HANDBOOK OF SPORTS MEDICINE

By Jason L. Dragoo, B.S.

Illustrations by Torey J. Arvik

RENAISSANCE PUBLISHING

Renaissance Publishing.
A division of *Renaissance Knowledge Systems, Inc.*

8634 S. Willow
Tempe, AZ 85284
(602) 820-0514

First Edition
Printed in the United States of America

Printing: 10 9 8 7 6 5 4 3 2 1

Publishers Cataloging in Publication Data

Dragoo, Jason L.
Handbook of Sports Medicine.

Includes bibliographical references.
Includes Index.
1. Sports medicine. 2. Athletic injuries. 3. Coaching—Preparation—Liability.
4. Injury prevention. I. Title.
Library of Congress Catalog Card Number 93-92722
ISBN 0-9637144-0-6

Dedication

Dedicated to all the coaches who volunteer their time for the benefit of others.

Contents

Foreword

Due to the physical nature of sports, injuries are all too common. Experts acknowledge that proper conditioning prior to participation is important in injury prevention, however, most youth sport organizations lack such programs. Too often, young athletes approach conditioning in a cavalier manner, assuming they are "in good shape" from running and playing with their friends. Some coaches simply have players "go through the motions" of stretching for a few minutes without supervision, while others do not bother with stretching at all to preserve valuable practice time. This text shows how conditioning can reduce injuries as well as hasten recovery time in many situations.

If an injury occurs, a trainer--if the athlete is fortunate enough to have one--or a coach is usually the first to see the harmed player. Whether the problem is minor or serious, it is imperative that the person in charge has at least a basic knowledge of treating the problem. With minor injuries, such understanding can minimize the amount of time an athlete sits on the sidelines. With major injuries, even knowing to not move the athlete and being prepared to rapidly request emergency medical care could mean the difference between life and death.

Although this book is not intended to make the reader an authority in Sports Medicine, its thoughtful use provides an excellent starting point for reducing the number and severity of sports injuries.

Thomas R. Carter, M.D.
Orthopedic Surgeon
Arizona State University

Preface

Each year, as many as 18 million people are hurt in the United States because of their participation in sports. According to hospital emergency room, doctors' and certified athletic trainers' records, 12 million people under 18 will sustain some type of permanent disability from sports *each year*. A quarter-million of these will be serious injuries such as spleen, liver or kidney problems, not to mention innumerable osteo-arthritis and other musculo-skeletal dysfunctions.

Participation in any sport brings with it occasional injuries. Statistics show that one in four amateur athletes will be injured during the season. Each year, 800,000 injuries and as many as 30 deaths occur in football alone, making it the most hazardous sport in the United States. The real tragedy is that 50% of these injuries could have been prevented.

It is time that we, as coaches, parents and athletes, address the fact that this is an epidemic that needs immediate attention. Whether we are volunteers or paid staff, we must take a hard look at our legal and professional liabilities. As a general rule, coaches and other professionals should take all possible steps to clear themselves from liability and to prepare themselves for unexpected events. It is the coach's duty to try to prevent injuries as well as know what to do should an injury occur. Coaches are not responsible for treating injuries, but they must have an emergency action plan ready in case an injury does occur.

As a physical therapist and certified athletic trainer for more than 19 years, I have seen the need for the development of effective Sports Medicine programs to help coaches, parents and the athletes themselves recognize, prevent and treat the inherent problem of sports: injuries. I feel that this text, developed by Jason Dragoo, is an excellent beginning in filling this need.

Bruce S. McCall, R.P.T., A.T.C.
Registered Physical Therapist
Certified Athletic Trainer

Acknowledgements

I gratefully and sincerely convey my appreciation to the following individuals for their contributions to this work:

My father, Mick, for his guidance and commitment to excellence in medicine and athletics, which was largely responsible for my interest in Sports Medicine and was instrumental in my success as a student-athlete. His dedication and motivation inspired the creation of this text.

My mother, Mary, for her love, compassion and friendship, not to mention her generosity in typing the seemingly endless drafts of this manuscript.

My brother, Justin, for his constant support and encouragement.

Jennifer, Amy and all my special friends. Without their priceless companionship and love, my efforts would have fallen far short of this goal.

Torey J. Arvik, illustrator, for his friendship and masterful artistic contributions, which have been instrumental in the success of this book.

Dr. Thomas Carter, M.D., and Bruce McCall, R.P.T., A.T.C., for their valuable guidance, support and clinical knowledge.

The professors in the School of Science and Math at California Polytechnic State University, San Luis Obispo, for their commitment to academic excellence.

Mary Westheimer for her expertise and editorial professionalism.

Mark Woodruff for his creative cover art.

To my colleagues and family members who gave invaluable assistance and support.

Jason L. Dragoo

Introduction

Whether working with athletes in community, recreational or school sport programs, coaches are often the unsung heroes of athletics. Coaches help athletes develop the confidence, inspiration and leadership skills that make athletic participation meaningful.

Even though these sports programs often operate with limited budgets, minimal equipment and modest medical expertise, their leaders understand that young athletes deserve the best care possible. That knowledge led to the development of this Sports Medicine text, which covers the prevention, recognition and treatment of sports injuries.

With its comprehensive coverage, coaches will want to have the *Handbook of Sports Medicine* with them at all times, including practice sessions (where most injuries occur) so they are best able to prevent or minimize problems. Unit 1 includes background information that *all* coaches should know. This unit should be read in its entirety and then re-read at the beginning of each competitive season. Unit 2 serves as a medical reference, with information about conditions that affect the entire body, conditions that apply to specific parts of the body and, finally, the best ways to prevent and treat these currently all-too-common situations. Coaches should become familiar with this unit's contents as well, so they are able to turn to the appropriate information in an emergency. When need arises, readers can refer to the **Quick Reference Injury Guide** inside the front cover, which directs coaches to the proper section for assistance. The index also helps coaches and athletes cross-reference information.

It is important to note, however, that this text is designed to give coaches and parents a *basic* level of Sports Medicine knowledge. If there is ever any doubt about the extent of injury or proper conditioning methods, please consult a medical professional. *This book in NO WAY replaces necessary medical care and should only be used as a guide to safely prepare athletes for competition and to prevent further harm should an injury occur.*

Regardless, we hope *Handbook of Sports Medicine* helps those dedicated individuals whom athletes call "Coach" to perform their services with greater ease and confidence than ever before.

Disclaimer

The information in this book is true and complete to the best of the author's knowledge. All recommendations are made without guarantee by the author. The purpose of this book is to educate coaches, athletes and parents in the basic principles of Sports Medicine. This text should be used only as a general guide and not an ultimate source of medical information. It is in *NO WAY* intended to educate anyone to treat injuries. Therefore, you should *always* consult a medical professional for proper guidance specific to your situation. The author and Renaissance Publishing are neither liable nor responsible to any person or entity with respect to any harm caused, or alleged to be caused, directly or indirectly by the information contained in this book.

If you do not wish to be bound by the above, you may return this book to the publisher for a full refund.

UNIT 1

THE FOUNDATION OF SPORTS MEDICINE

This first unit provides the background every coach and athlete needs to excel. You will learn more about how your body works, how to approach problems should they arise, and how to achieve success through fitness in mind and body.

These four chapters give you the foundation you need to use Unit 2 effectively, so please read and study them thoroughly.

1 The Basics

Without a solid foundation in human body dynamics, trying to be the best coach or athlete you can be is like trying to win a championship without ever practicing. This first chapter helps you better grasp how and why the human body works. Reading this section first will help you perform at your highest level for years to come.

1.1 SPORTS MEDICINE TERMINOLOGY

If you understand standard terminology, you can better communicate with medical professionals in emergency situations. Learning these terms will also help you better grasp certain procedures necessary for recognizing and treating sports injuries.

The glossary explains general terms, and the General Anatomy and Physiology section then provides the names of the body parts and processes while showing how they all work together.

A

ABC Method- The sequence of operations for cardiopulmonary resuscitation: **A**-airway, **B**-breathing, **C**-circulation.

Abduction- Movement of a body part *away from* the midline of the body. (see Adduction and Circumduction)

Abrasion- A superficial wound in which the upper layer of skin is scraped off.

Acclimatization- The adjustment of the body to a new environment.

Acute- Recent.

Adduction- Movement of a body part *toward* the midline of the body. (see Abduction and Circumduction)

Analgesic- A pain relieving agent.

Anatomy-	The study of human body structure and form.
Anesthetic-	An agent that produces general or local numbness and insensibility to pain, stimulation or touch.
Anterior-	The front of the body, or front body part. (see Posterior)
Anti-inflammatory-	A drug that reduces swelling.
Antipyretic-	A fever-reducing drug.
Antiseptic-	An agent that stops the growth of microorganisms.
Atrophy-	Decrease in tissue or muscle size.
Avulsion-	An injury that leaves a piece of skin torn from its original position.

B

Brachial Artery-	The main artery of the arm.

C

Calcium-	A mineral element found in the body that is important for proper fluid balance and muscle activity.
Calisthenics-	Exercises that use the body's weight to improve muscular strength and endurance.
Cardiovascular-	Pertaining to the heart and blood vessels.
Cartilage-	Gristle-like padding on or between bones at a joint.
Cervical-	Pertaining to the neck; seven vertebrae in neck region.
Chlorine-	A molecule found in the body that functions as an electrolyte.
Chronic-	The opposite of acute; drawn out or recurring.

Circumduction- Any circular motion of the shoulder or hip joint. (see Abduction and Adduction)

Compound Fracture- A fracture in which bones penetrate the surfaces of skin. Also called an open fracture.

Concussion- A mild state of disorientation or temporary unconsciousness caused by a blow to the head.

Contraction- Shortening of muscle fibers.

Contusion- An injury in which the skin is not broken, but capillaries are ruptured; a bruise. The discoloration is caused by internal bleeding.

Cranial- Pertaining to the skull or head region.

Cruciate Ligament- A connective tissue in knee joints that give the knees anterior-posterior stability.

Cryokinetics- Treatment using cold and movement.

Cryotherapy- Use of cold, such as ice, as treatment.

Cyanosis- Blue or gray skin color caused by oxygen deficiency in the blood.

D

Diastolic Pressure- Pressure exerted on the internal walls of the arteries when the heart is relaxing.

Dilate- To enlarge or widen.

Dislocation- Complete displacement of a joint.

Distal- Farther from the heart, when compared to something closer to the heart. The opposite of Proximal.

Dorsal- The back surface or back. The opposite of Ventral.

Dorsiflexion- Upward movement of a body part from normal position.

Dyspnea- Labored or difficult breathing.

E

Edema- Swelling; accumulation of fluid in tissues or cavities.

Electrolyte- Molecules responsible for conduction of electrical charges. These include potassium, sodium, and chlorine.

Enzyme- A protein that accelerates chemical reactions.

Erythema- Reddening of the skin.

F

Femoral Artery- The main artery supplying the thigh and leg.

Flaccid- Soft, limp.

Flexion- The act of bending or condition of being bent; in contrast to extension.

Fracture- A break, crack or crumbling of a bone.

G

Good Samaritan Laws- A series of laws written to protect emergency care personnel. These laws require anyone providing assistance to maintain a standard of care in good faith within the provider's level of training and best ability.

Greenstick Fracture - An incomplete fracture.

H

Heat Cramps - A condition brought on by the loss of body fluids. Common in hot environments when perspiring.

Heat Exhaustion- A condition in which blood pools in the vessels of the skin because the body is trying to dispel excessive heat.

Heat Stroke- Failure of the body's heat regulating mechanisms.

Hematoma- The collection of blood under the skin or in the tissues after a blood vessel has broken.

Hemorrhage- Internal or external bleeding.

Hydrotherapy- Treatment by use of water.

Hyperthermia- Extremely high body temperature.

Hyperventilation- A condition that results in carbon dioxide deficiency in the blood; caused by increased rate and decreased depth of breathing.

Hypothermia- Low body temperature.

I

Innervate- To stimulate a nerve or body part.

Isokinetic- Exercise in which maximum, constant resistance is provided through the full range movement.

Isometric-	The contraction of a muscle without body movement or shortening of the muscle fibers. Builds static strength.
Isotonic-	The contraction of a muscle in which the muscle fibers shorten and cause movement of the adjoining body parts.

K

Kinesiology-	Study of human movement.

L

Lateral-	Away from the midline of the body, toward the side. (see Medial)
Ligament-	Semi-elastic, tough connective tissue that connects bone to bone.

M

Mechanism of Injury-	How the injury occurred.
Medial-	Toward the midline of the body. (see Lateral)
Modality-	An apparatus or method of therapy used in rehabilitation.
Myositis-	Inflammation of muscle.
Myositis Ossificans-	Bone formation in muscle tissue caused from a chronic contusion or hematoma.

O

Ossification- The process of bone formation.

P

Palpation- Examination by touch.

Physiology- A branch of biology that deals with the functions and activities of living matter.

Plantarflexion- Downward movement of the foot.

Point Tenderness- Tenderness caused by pressure over a particular spot.

Posterior- The back of the body or back body part. (see Anterior)

Potassium- An element found in the body that acts as an electrolyte. Important for proper fluid balance and muscle activity.

Pressure Point- Areas for exerting pressure to control bleeding.

Proximal- Closer to a point of reference (usually the heart). The opposite of Distal; closer to the heart.

Pulse- Expansion and contraction of arterial walls as the heart pumps blood.

R

Radial Pulse- Wrist pulse.

Range of Motion- The amount of movement about a given joint.

Romberg Sign- A test to indicate neuro-cranial disturbance. The body's inability to maintain balance when eyes are closed and feet are placed together indicate a neuro-cranial problem.

S

Shock- Failure of the circulatory system to provide an adequate blood supply to all parts of the body.

Sign- Any bodily manifestation that serves to indicate the presence of a disorder.

Sodium- An element found in the body that acts as an electrolyte. Sodium is important for proper fluid balance and muscle activity.

Splint- Any device that will immobilize a body part.

Sprain- An injury in which ligaments are excessively stretched or torn.

Stimulant- An agent that temporarily increases functional activity.

Strain- An injury in which muscles or tendons are excessively stretched or torn.

Subluxation- Partial dislocation.

Symptom- Any phenomenon that is a departure from normal function.

Systolic Pressure- Force exerted by the blood on the arterial walls when the heart is contracting.

T

Tendon- Tough tissue that connects muscle to bone.

Thermotherapy- Treatment with heat.

Torque- A rotary force.

Trauma- Physical or mental injury.

V

Vascular- Pertaining to or composed of blood vessels.

Vasoconstriction- Blood vessel constriction.

Vasodilation- Blood vessel dilation.

Ventral- Bottom surface, belly. Opposite of Dorsal.

Vital Signs- Pulse rate, breathing rate, blood pressure and relative skin temperature.

1.2 ANATOMY AND PHYSIOLOGY

Our bodies are a complex network of systems that complement each other to achieve a great variety of movements and functions that are unique to humans.

The smallest functional unit of the body is the **cell**. It is capable of growth, movement and reproduction. Cells form specialized groups that are called **tissues**. Groups of tissues create **organs** that, in turn, join to form the seven main **organ systems**.

These seven systems are the:

- •Circulatory system
- •Nervous system

- Respiratory system
- Digestive system
- Endocrine system
- Urogenital system
- Musculo-skeletal system.

CIRCULATORY SYSTEM

The circulatory system takes nutrients and oxygen to all body tissues as well as removes carbon dioxide and other metabolic wastes. The **heart** is a specialized muscle that circulates the blood. Humans have a four-chambered heart composed of two **atria** and two **ventricles**, which are separated by a **septum** (figure 1-1). The heart also has four main valves to prevent the back flow of blood. The normal route of blood flow is:

HEART > ARTERIES > ARTERIOLES > CAPILLARIES > VENULES > VEINS > HEART.

Arteries are vessels that take blood *away* from the heart, while **veins** bring blood *back* to the heart. **Capillaries** are vessels in which the blood and tissues exchange

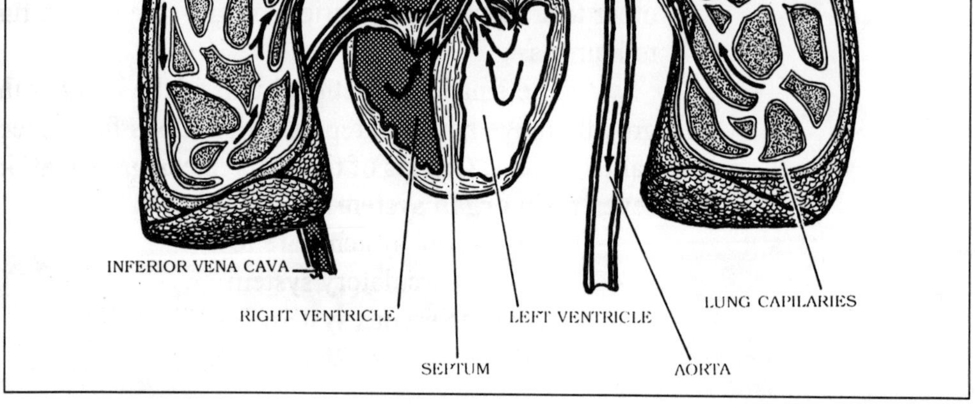

figure 1-1. Blood flow in the heart and lungs. Shaded vessels indicate blood is deoxygenated. Clear vessels represent blood that has been reoxygenated by the lungs.

nutrients and wastes. Blood is expelled from the heart with considerable force that creates a higher blood pressure (force against the walls of the arteries) than the blood traveling through the veins. The pressure caused by heart contraction is **systolic pressure**. The residual pressure in the arteries when the heart is relaxed is **diastolic pressure**. These two pressures comprise the blood pressure measurement which is always read as:

$^{systolic}/_{diastolic}$ (for example, $^{120}/_{80}$).

Blood, the circulating medium, is composed of many structures, primarily red blood cells, white blood cells, plasma, nutrients, hormones and assorted other proteins. **Red blood cells**, which are made in bone marrow, contain **hemoglobin**, which carries oxygen to the cells and carbon dioxide to the lungs. **White blood cells** attack intruding bacteria and other foreign objects and thereby help prevent infections. **Plasma** is the liquid part of the blood in which all the solid elements are suspended.

The **lymphatic system** works intimately with the circulatory system. It helps the white blood cells with the defense process and also circulates certain nutrients. White blood cells and other defenders trap foreign bodies in networks of tubes called **lymph nodes**.

NERVOUS SYSTEM

The nervous system either directly or indirectly controls all other systems of the body. Its main functions include maintaining a constant internal environment and adapting the body to changing external conditions.

The nervous system can be divided into two main parts:

- The **central nervous system (CNS)**, which consists of the brain and the spinal column
- The **peripheral nervous system (PNS)**, which consists of the paired spinal nerves.

The system can be further divided into the **autonomic** (unconsciously controlled) system, which regulates the heart rate, and the **somatic** (or consciously controlled) system, which stimulates skeletal muscles.

The nervous system communicates externally through the sense organs such as the eyes and ears by sending messages through the **sensory nerves** and CNS to the brain for processing. The brain then sends information back through the CNS to the **motor nerves**, where they activate or inhibit body processes. Certain impulses, however, do not travel all the way to the brain. A message may travel up the sensory nerves to the spinal cord, and then directly back to the motor nerves, which end on **motor units**. These units lie directly on muscle fibers. This type of nervous response, known as a **reflex arc** (figure 1-2), is responsible for the kicking response when a doctor hits the tendon below the knee.

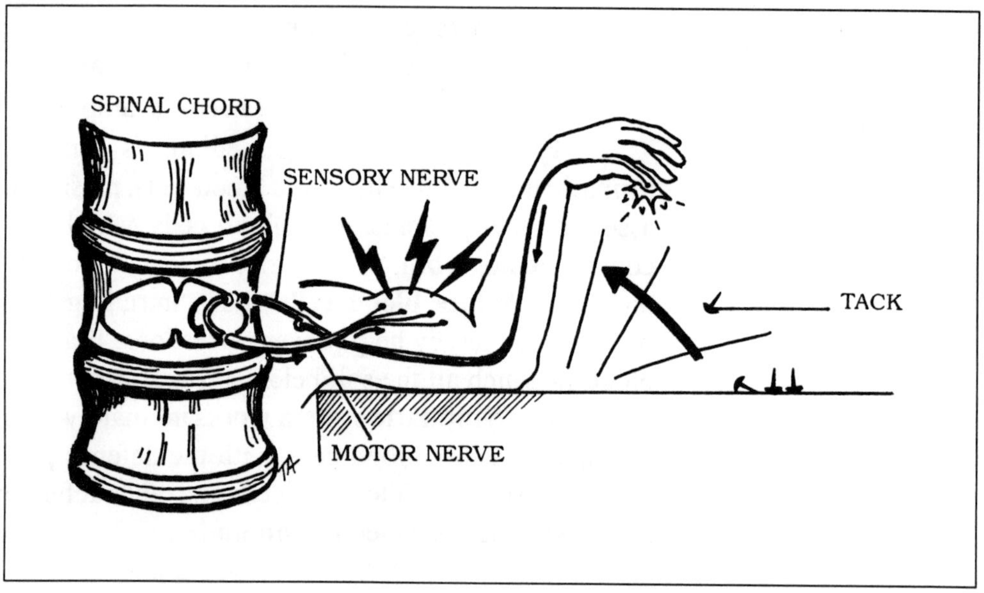

figure 1-2. A reflex arc. A sensory message of external harm (Tack) travels from nerves in the injured finger to the spinal cord. Here, the signal is quickly transferred to the motor nerves which activate the muscles (in this case the biceps) to pull the limb off the tack. During a reflex arc, signals do not reach the brain until after movement has been initiated.

RESPIRATORY SYSTEM

Every living cell in the human body requires **oxygen** for its metabolic processes and the generation of energy. Through the evolutionary process, our bodies have become extremely efficient at taking in oxygen from the environment and exhaling **carbon dioxide**, which is a waste product.

Air enters the body through the **nose** or **mouth**. The nasal cavity contains many blood vessels and is lined with mucous and small hairs called **cilia**. These allow the air to be filtered, warmed and saturated with water vapor. Foreign material filtered by the mucous is swept along to the **pharynx** where it can be expelled from the body by the coughing or sneezing reflex.

The cleansed, warmed air now passes down the **larynx**. This region contains the **vocal chords**, which are two pieces of tissue that vibrate at different frequencies when air is expelled from the lungs during speech. Larger foreign particles are filtered in this region as well, and are forcefully expelled by coughing. The larynx also contains the region where the **esophagus**, or food tube, and the **trachea**, or windpipe, separate food and air respectively. This is accomplished by the **epiglottis**, which seals off the trachea when food or liquid is swallowed.

figure 1-3. The repiratory system. Note that the microscopic alveoli, the air sacs where the blood exchanges carbon dioxide for oxygen, have been enlarged to show their structure.

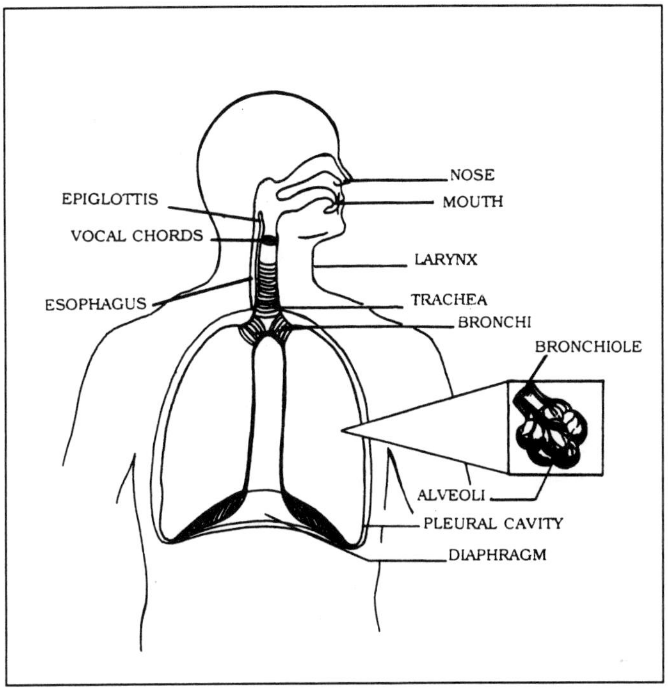

Air now passes down the **trachea**, which has cartilage rings that give the walls considerable structural integrity. Here, filtering mechanisms similar to those in the upper respiratory tract continue to eliminate unwanted particles. The trachea ends by dividing into two tubes, named **bronchi** (each is called a **bronchus**), which take air to the respective lungs. These bronchi further divide into many small **bronchioles** (figure 1-3).

The air passage ends in the **alveoli**, which are specialized pouches that allow gas to exchange with the blood. The tremendous surface area created by the 350 million alveoli facilitate the exchange.

Air is inhaled into the lungs by the downward contraction of the **diaphragm** and other respiratory muscles. The contraction creates negative pressure in the lung cavity compared to the outside air. The air is then exhaled passively when the respiratory muscles relax, increasing pressure in the lung cavity and forcing out air. During exercise, we exhale actively because our rib muscles help force air out quickly so we can take in more oxygen.

The lungs themselves are in the **pleural cavity**, a sealed, fluid-filled cavity that maintains a pressure consistently lower than that inside the lungs and thus prevents them from collapsing.

DIGESTIVE SYSTEM

It is easiest to understand the digestive system by following the path of ingested food. Food is first physically broken down by the **teeth**, which grind the material into a soft, swallowable mass. The salivary glands secret **saliva** that moistens the food and begins the chemical breakdown of **starch**, or complex sugars, by enzymes.

After swallowing, the food travels down the **esophagus** under the influence of **peristalsis**, the wave-like contraction of the muscles surrounding the esophagus that forces food and liquid into the stomach.

Food is further broken down into **chyme** by the physical grinding of the **stomach** walls and by the acidic chemical environment produced by cells in the stomach. **Hydrochloric acid** and a host of other enzymes are responsible for the break down of proteins and other food particles.

The acidic chyme now passes from the stomach into the first part of the small intestine, which is called the **duodenum**. Here, secretions of the **pancreas** neutralize the acid, and enzymes released from the **gall bladder** digest fats. Dozens of other enzymes in the duodenum essentially complete the digestion of proteins, fats and carbohydrates. The chyme then reaches the second and third parts of the small intestine, the **jejunum** and the **ileum**, respectively. This is

figure 1-4. The digestive system. Nutrients are first absorbed through the villi, then pass directly into the hepatic portal system where they are taken to the liver for processing.

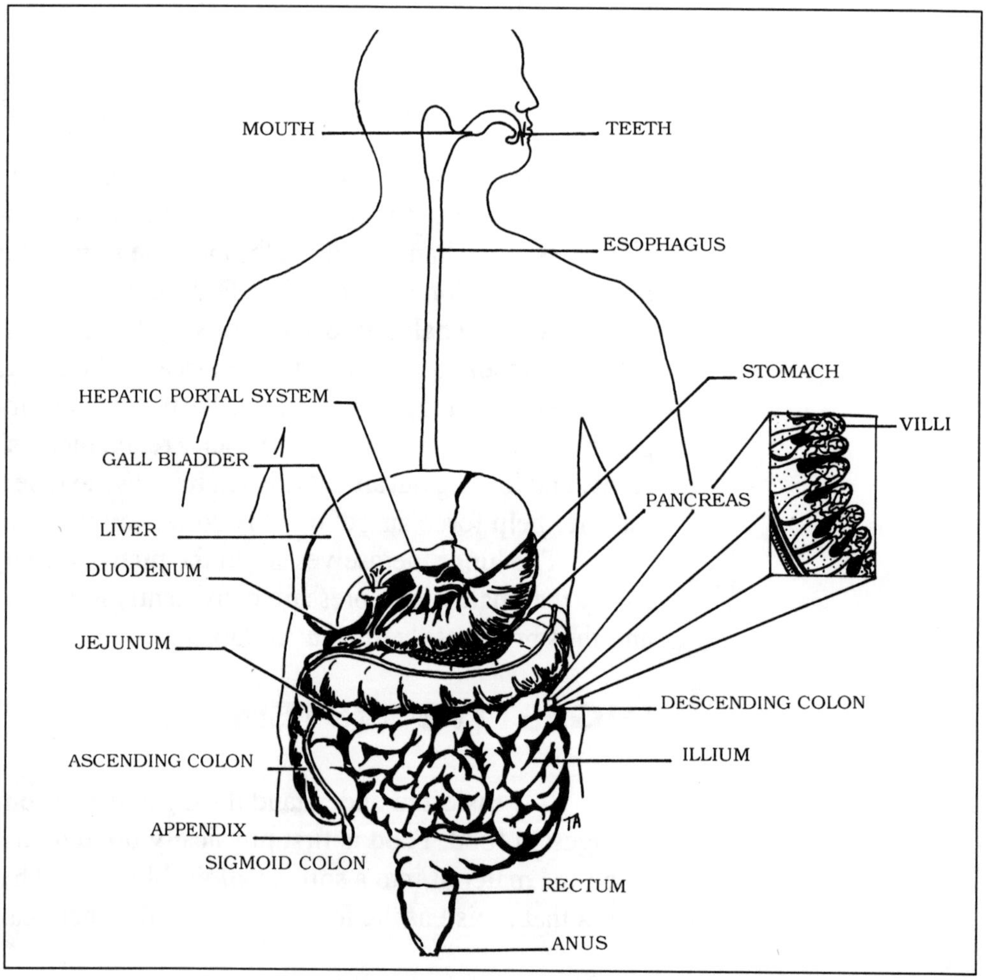

where most nutrients are absorbed through the **villi** (figure 1-4) in the intestinal wall.

The absorbed nutrients directly enter the blood and travel through the **hepatic portal system** of veins to the **liver**. The liver is the body's main chemical processing unit, where nutrients are stored and rearranged, bile is produced, and drugs and other poisons—including alcohol—are detoxified.

The nutrients that will be used directly for energy exist as **glucose**. As blood glucose levels increase, the pancreas excretes **insulin**, a hormone that allows blood sugar to be absorbed by various body tissues as **glycogen** and thereby lowers blood sugar levels. If there is not enough active insulin, a person develops **diabetes mellitis**, which must be controlled by a proper diet and sometimes even insulin injections (see section 2.6). If blood sugar levels are low, the pancreas secretes another hormone called **glucagon**, to accelerate glucose reabsorption into the bloodstream.

Any food that is not absorbed in the small intestine passes into the **large intestine**, or **colon**. Where the small intestine ends and the colon begins, there is a small remnant of a gland called the **appendix**. The appendix does not affect digestion and is usually removed when it becomes inflamed, a condition called appendicitis. The colon itself has four regions, **ascending**, **transverse**, **descending** and **sigmoid**.

These regions extract water and vitamins from undigested food, which is mostly fiber. When the colon becomes inflamed or diseased, water is not extracted as efficiently, producing diarrhea. Conversely, dehydration or a low-fiber diet creates a lack of moisture in the bowels, causing constipation.

The undigestible wastes are stored in the **rectum** until they leave the body through the **anus**.

ENDOCRINE SYSTEM

The **endocrine**, or ductless gland, system controls the other body systems. The gland secretions, or **hormones**, enter directly into the blood system and are circulated to every part of the body. Certain cells have receptors that recognize specific hormones which will directly influence the cell's activity. The major endocrine glands (figure 1-5) are:

- Pituitary
- Thyroid
- Parathyroid
- Pancreas
- Adrenal

•Testes
•Ovaries.

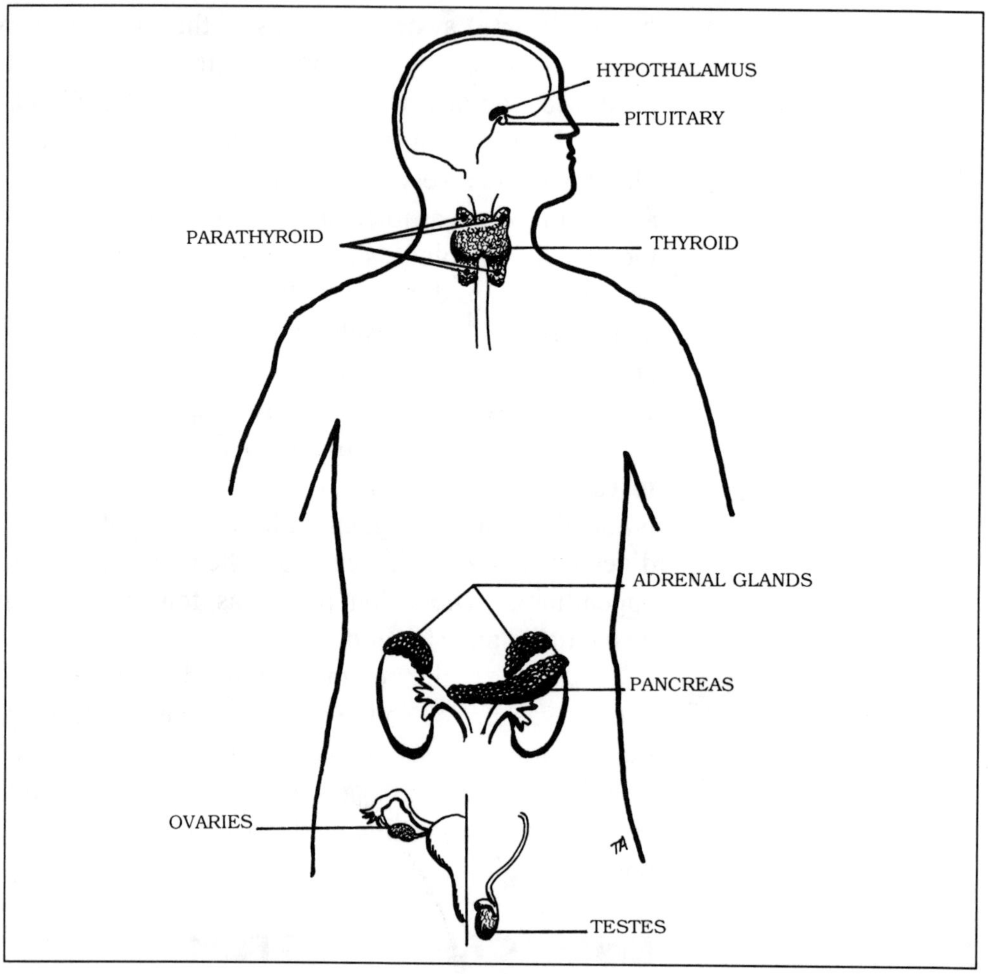

figure 1-5. The major endocrine glands. The hypothalamus, which is not an endocrine gland, is noted because of its intimate role with this system.

In the base of the brain is the **pituitary gland**, which is often referred to as "the master gland" because it controls many body processes. Now, however, recent studies suggest that the **hypothalamus**, which is also found in the brain, regulates the pituitary, prompting many specialists to call the hypothalamus the master gland. The pituitary is comprised of two main regions: the anterior and posterior. The anterior pituitary secretes **growth hormone -GH-**, which is necessary for normal bone and muscle growth and development, **thyrotropin -TSH-**, which stimulates the thyroid, **adrenocorticotropin -ACTH-**, which stimulates the adrenal gland, **prolactin -LTH-**, which serves a variety of functions in the reproductive system, and **follicle stimulating hormone -FSH-** and **luteinizing hormone -LH-**, which are responsible for sperm and egg development as well as secretion of the sex hormones (which are further discussed in the section on testes and ovaries). The posterior pituitary secretes **vasopressin**, also called **anti-diuretic hormone -ADH-**, which is responsible for water reabsorption in the kidneys, and **oxytocin**, which stimulates the pregnant uterus and mammary tissue.

The **thyroid**, which is located in the neck, secretes **thyroxin**, which controls the **basal metabolic rate (BMR)**, the rate at which cells **respire**, or burn energy. BMR is important in athletics and weight loss and is discussed later in the text. The thyroid also produces **calcitonin**, which increases the uptake of calcium into the bones.

As figure 1-5 shows, the four **parathyroid glands** are near the thyroid. They excrete **parathyroid hormone**, which opposes the effect of calcitonin, therefore increasing calcium uptake from the bones into the blood.

In addition to other digestive enzymes, the pancreas, located below the stomach, produces two main hormones, insulin and glucagon, which were covered in the section on digestion.

Directly on top of the kidneys are the **adrenal glands**, which have an outer cortex region and an inner medulla region. The **cortex** produces three main hormones: **cortisol**, which regulates carbohydrate metabolism, **aldosterone**, which increases sodium retention in the kidneys, and small amounts of sex hormones such as testosterone and estrogen. The **medulla** produces **epinephrine**, or adrenaline, and **norepinephrine**, which are important in the "flight or fright" defense process.

The **gonads**, or **testes and ovaries**, determine the primary and secondary sex characteristics of males and females. The testes produce **testosterone**, which is responsible for sperm production, male growth and development patterns, and secondary sex characteristics such as facial hair and the deepening of the voice. Ovaries produce **estrogen** and **progesterone**, which are necessary for ovule formation, menstruation, maintenance of pregnancy, development of female anatomy and secondary sex characteristics such as enlargement of the mammary glands. Both males and females produce all the sex hormones, but one group is produced in a much greater amount, thereby directing sexual development.

UROGENITAL SYSTEM

The urogenital system filters wastes from the circulatory system. This system also contains the organs of copulation, more specifically the penis and vagina.

The **kidneys** are the body's primary filter. The kidneys have an extensive vascular network that enables them to completely filter all the blood in a body every four minutes.

Blood is carried to a highly convoluted capillary bed, called the **glomerulus**, which is surrounded by a thin membrane called **Bowman's capsule**. Wastes, ions and small nutrient molecules diffuse across the capillary walls into Bowman's capsule and then into the convoluted tubule system (figure 1-6). Here, nutrients and water are reabsorbed into the blood, and the waste, mainly composed of **urea** (a by-product of protein metabolism) and surplus ions, is concentrated into urine. The **urine** is fed through the **collecting duct system** into the **renal pelvis** (figure 1-7), then passed into the **ureters** and down into the **urinary bladder** by rhythmic contractions (peristalsis). The urine is stored in the bladder until eliminated through the **urethra**.

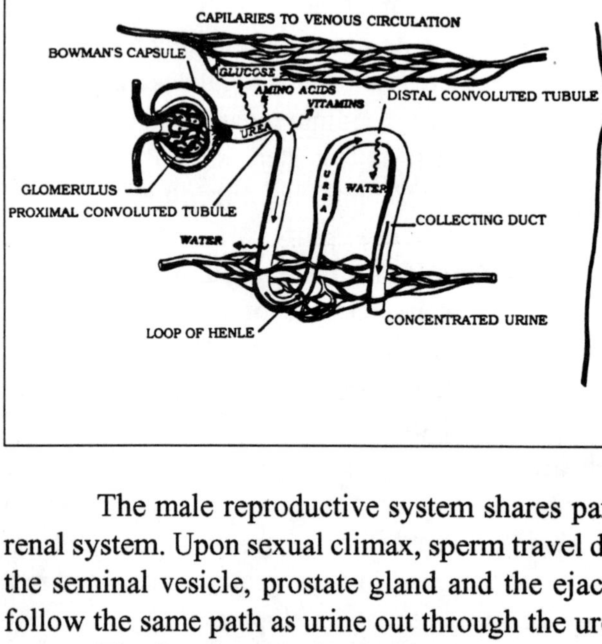

figure 1-6. The convoluted tubule system of the kidney. Blood filters through the glomerulus where wastes and nutrients are transfered into the tubule system. Nutrients are drawn back into the surrounding capillaries, while wastes are concentrated into urine.

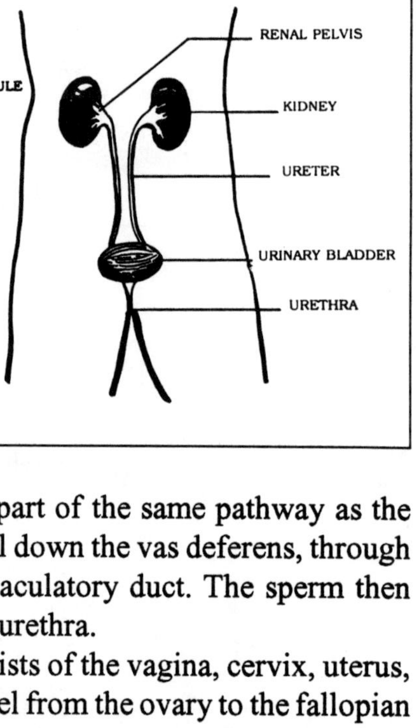

figure 1-7. The urinary system. Urine passes from the kidneys, down the ureters, to the bladder where it is stored until elimination through the urethra.

The male reproductive system shares part of the same pathway as the renal system. Upon sexual climax, sperm travel down the vas deferens, through the seminal vesicle, prostate gland and the ejaculatory duct. The sperm then follow the same path as urine out through the urethra.

The female reproductive anatomy consists of the vagina, cervix, uterus, fallopian tubes and ovaries. Mature ovules travel from the ovary to the fallopian tubes (which are not connected to each other) for fertilization. Sperm must contact the egg in the first third of the fallopian tube to achieve pregnancy. Whether fertilized or unfertilized, the egg travels to the uterus. If the egg is fertilized, it implants into the uterus wall. If the egg is unfertilized, it is expelled during menstruation.

MUSCULO-SKELETAL SYSTEM

Skeletal System

A thorough understanding of the skeletal system, which is comprised of the bones and their corresponding connective tissues, and its intimate relationship with the muscular system is essential in the study of Sports Medicine. The skeletal system serves many functions including:

- The protection of vital organs
- The support of soft tissues
- The production of blood cells in the soft, pulpy bone marrow
- Serving as a reservoir for minerals (calcium and phosphorus)
- Serving as a system of levers to receive torque from the muscles, which produce movement.

Bone itself is made of mineral and organic components that create its characteristic hard consistency, which is comparable to the strength of iron. The 208 bones of the human body can be divided into two main groups: the axial skeleton and the appendicular skeleton.

The **axial skeleton** contains the skull, thorax (or rib cage), pelvis and vertebral column (or spine). The **skull** contains 29 bones that are fused to form a protective casing for the brain. The movable **mandible**, or jawbone, is also included here. The thorax contains 25 bones that include the 12 pairs of **ribs** and the **sternum**, or breastbone. The **pelvis** is comprised of the two large **illiac**, or hip, bones and the other fused bones that form the hip girdle. The **vertebral column** consists of 33 bones that can be divided into five regions: the **cervical** spine (seven bones in the neck), **thoracic** spine (12 bones), **lumbar** spine (five bones in the lower back), the **sacrum** (five fused bones in the hip region) and the **coccyx** (four bones that comprise the tailbone). The axial skeleton is responsible for erect posture as well as providing a relatively stable base for the attachment of muscles moving the appendicular skeleton.

The **appendicular skeleton** contains the extremities. The upper right and left extremities, which we commonly call arms, begin anatomically with the shoulder girdle and end with the fingertips. The lower extremities, which we call legs, begin anatomically at the hip joint and end at the toes.

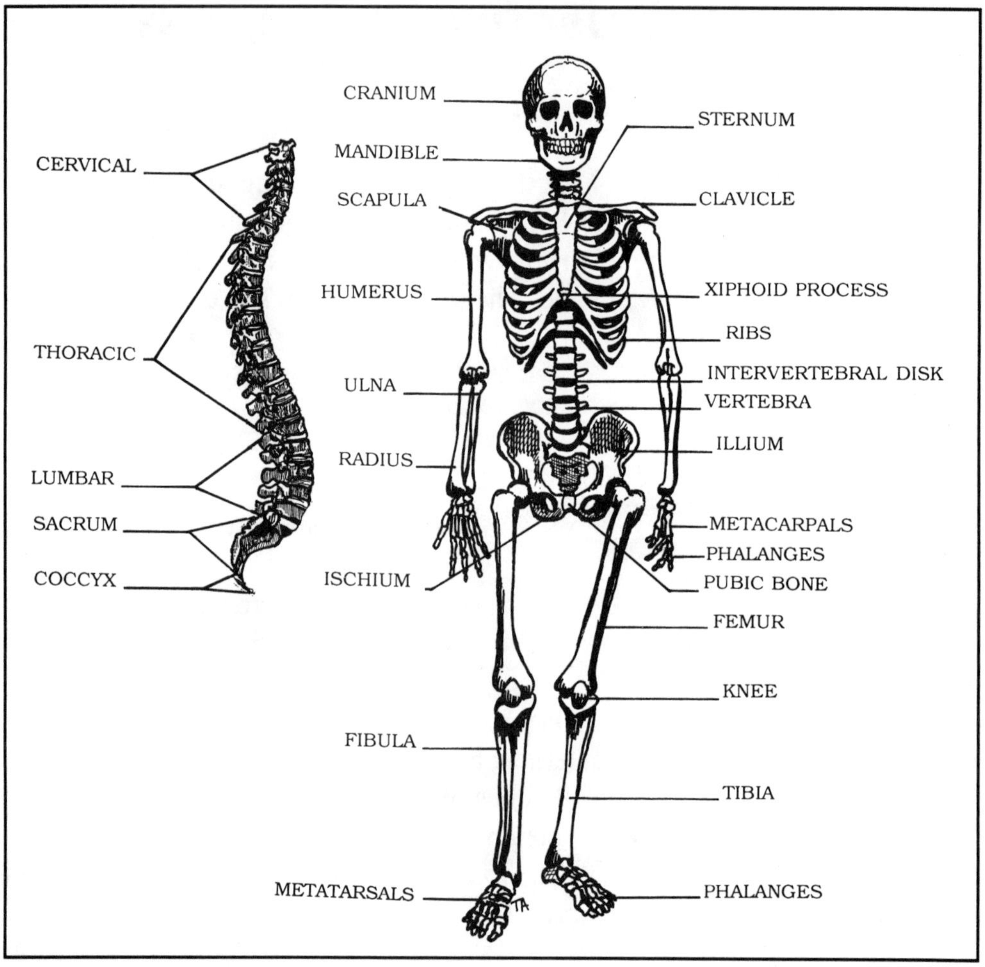

figure 1-8. The human skeleton. Readers should be familiar with the names and positions of all bones listed.

Bones join to form a series of moveable segments that are responsible for the wide range of human movements. The junction between two bones is an **articulation**, or **joint**. Moveable articulations are held together by **ligaments**, which are tough, relatively elastic, gristle-like tissues that connect bone to bone. Ligaments should not be confused with **tendons**, which have many of the same physical properties but connect *muscle* to bone.

The joints' articulating surfaces are covered with **cartilage** that provides a frictionless surface to facilitate movement. Even though cartilage is tough, bendable and capable of absorbing a considerable amount of shock, its surface can become roughened and torn. This degeneration of the articular cartilage is called **chondromalacia**. Cartilage's regeneration ability is limited, which makes chondromalacia all too common in athletes who overtrain.

Joints are entirely encased in **capsules** that house **synovial fluid** (figure 1-9). This viscous fluid lubricates and nourishes the cartilage. Movement stimulates the production of synovial fluid. Exercise also changes the consistency of the fluid to allow a greater range of joint motion and increased cartilage nourishment. Understanding these effects make it easy to see why warm-up exercises are so important for athletic competition.

Finally, the bones themselves are varied in form and function. **Long bones**, such as the **femur**, or thigh, and **humerus**, or upper arm, act as levers when moved by the skeletal muscles. Generally, the bones of the lower extremities are larger and stronger because they receive the repeated stress of weight bearing. **Short bones**, such as the fingers and vertebrae, provide a greater range of motion and shock absorption. **Flat bones**, found in the skull and sternum, protect the vital organs and provide a broad surface for muscle attachment. **Irregular bones** are shaped specifically to provide passageways for nerves, vessels and ducts.

Now that you know the purpose of these various types of bones, if someone handed you one, you could presume much about its function just

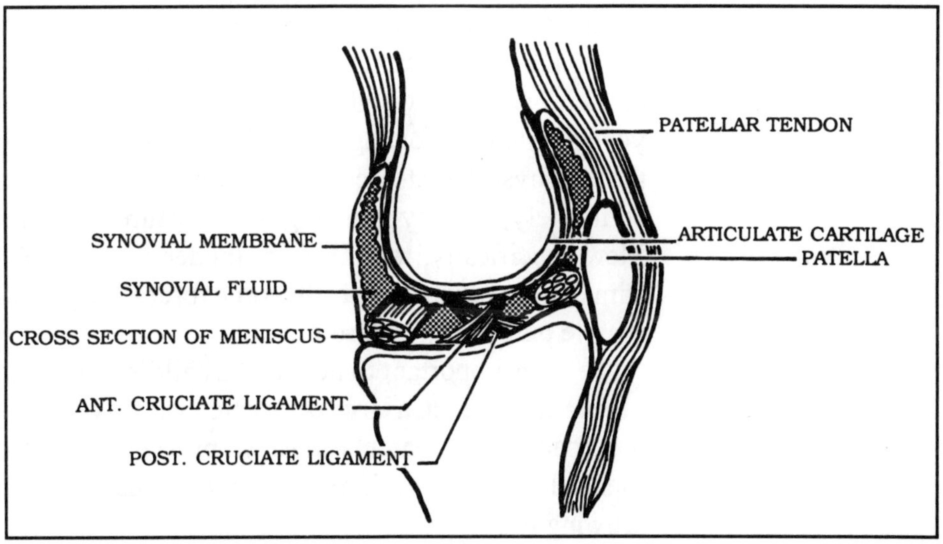

figure 1-9. A cross-section of an articulation (joint). The shaded area represents synovial fluid which is encased by the synovial membrane.

from its size and shape. Such knowledge is especially important for coaches and athletes. We recommend studying and learning the names and positions of the major bones of the human skeleton shown in figure 1-8.

Although bone contains a large amount of lifeless minerals, it is considered a living tissue. Most bones grow from a region called the **epiphysis**, which contains the **epiphyseal plates**. These plates are composed of cartilage that grows and turns into bone, or **ossifies**, as we progress from childhood to the end of puberty. We will talk more about this process at the end of this section.

Besides this growth process, specialized cells constantly remodel bone tissue to accommodate external stresses. This remodeling has important implications in training. For example, if a young pitcher constantly exercised only one arm, then the bone will grow and develop in a slightly different internal configuration than the relatively unstressed bones of the opposite arm. This shows the importance of the **uniform** (or **symmetrical**) **training principle**, in which both sides of the body should be exposed to the same amount of external force to maintain muscle and bone symmetry, and equal range of motion. The pitcher's training regime, then, also should include weight training exercises for the unexercised arm to maintain equal strength.

Careful, well-balanced training is essential for young athletes. Their skeletal system is growing rapidly, so training techniques during adolescence can directly alter a child's permanent bone configuration. Obviously, understanding and using proper physiological principles is imperative when working with youngsters.

Children who start early in athletic activities, especially in sports like gymnastics that require specialized movements, seem to especially excel. Still, during these early stages, muscles and bones should only be exposed to the stress of their own body weight. Unsupervised weight training is *not* appropriate for young athletes before age 14 or 15 (see section 3.5) because excessive stress on the epiphyseal plates can wear down and chip cartilage or even pull it off completely, thereby inducing plate closure and arresting further bone growth. More specifically, tension from moderate (athlete's body weight) muscle pull stimulates growth, while shearing forces, compression, impact, or excessive muscle pull tend to retard growth.

It is important to note that a child's size is not a good indication of bone maturation. In fact, a large child often will have very immature bones. Overzealous coaches and parents must be prevented from overtraining such athletes, especially since their large body weight usually maximally stresses their fast-growing tissues.

So remember, exercise and non-traumatic stress enhances bone and muscle growth and strength. For prepubescent athletes, heavy weight training and overtraining can damage cartilage and arrest bone growth. Moderation is the key to training youngsters. Let them grow into their bodies by teaching them agility and coordination, while exercising their minds.

Muscular System

Muscle tissue serves many functions in the human body. Even though their structure and function varies considerably, muscles have four common properties: **irritability**, **contractibility**, **distensibility** and **elasticity**.

Irritability refers to the ability to be stimulated by electrical impulses from the nervous system. Contractibility identifies muscles' abilities to shorten in relation to its resting length. Distensibility refers to the ability to be stretched beyond resting length, and elasticity refers to the capacity to recoil, or return to its original shape and length.

There are three muscle types in humans:

•Smooth
•Cardiac
•Striated, or skeletal.

Smooth muscle is characterized by involuntary spindle shaped cells. They surround the digestive tract, vessels and other organs controlled by the autonomic nervous system. Their job is to maintain **homeostasis**, or a constant internal environment, by transporting materials via peristalsis. Smooth muscles also are vital in other regulatory systems.

Cardiac muscle is only found in the heart and has the unique ability to contract without nervous stimulation, a property called **autorhythmicity**. Cardiac muscle also is extensively branched, allowing conduction of impulses from one cell to another.

Striated muscles are the voluntary muscles responsible for human movement, and therefore are the focus of this section.

We have approximately 500 voluntary muscles in our bodies, and they must receive conscious direction from the nervous system. Skeletal muscle serves many functions including:

•Supplying the force needed to move body parts
•Resisting movement of a body part
•Supplying force needed to stabilize body parts.

To accomplish these functions, striated muscle is capable of three types of contractions. **Isometric** contractions do not result in a change of muscle length. In other words, there is no movement of body parts, so this is sometimes called a static contraction. For instance, contracting the quadriceps, or thigh muscles, while standing is an isometric contraction. Notice that the muscles do not move the lower leg because there is no change in muscle length. This contraction can be accomplished at all joint angles as long as a constant muscle length is kept. **Isotonic** contraction involves a change of figure 1-10. The muscular system. Readers should be familiar with the names and positions of all muscles shown.

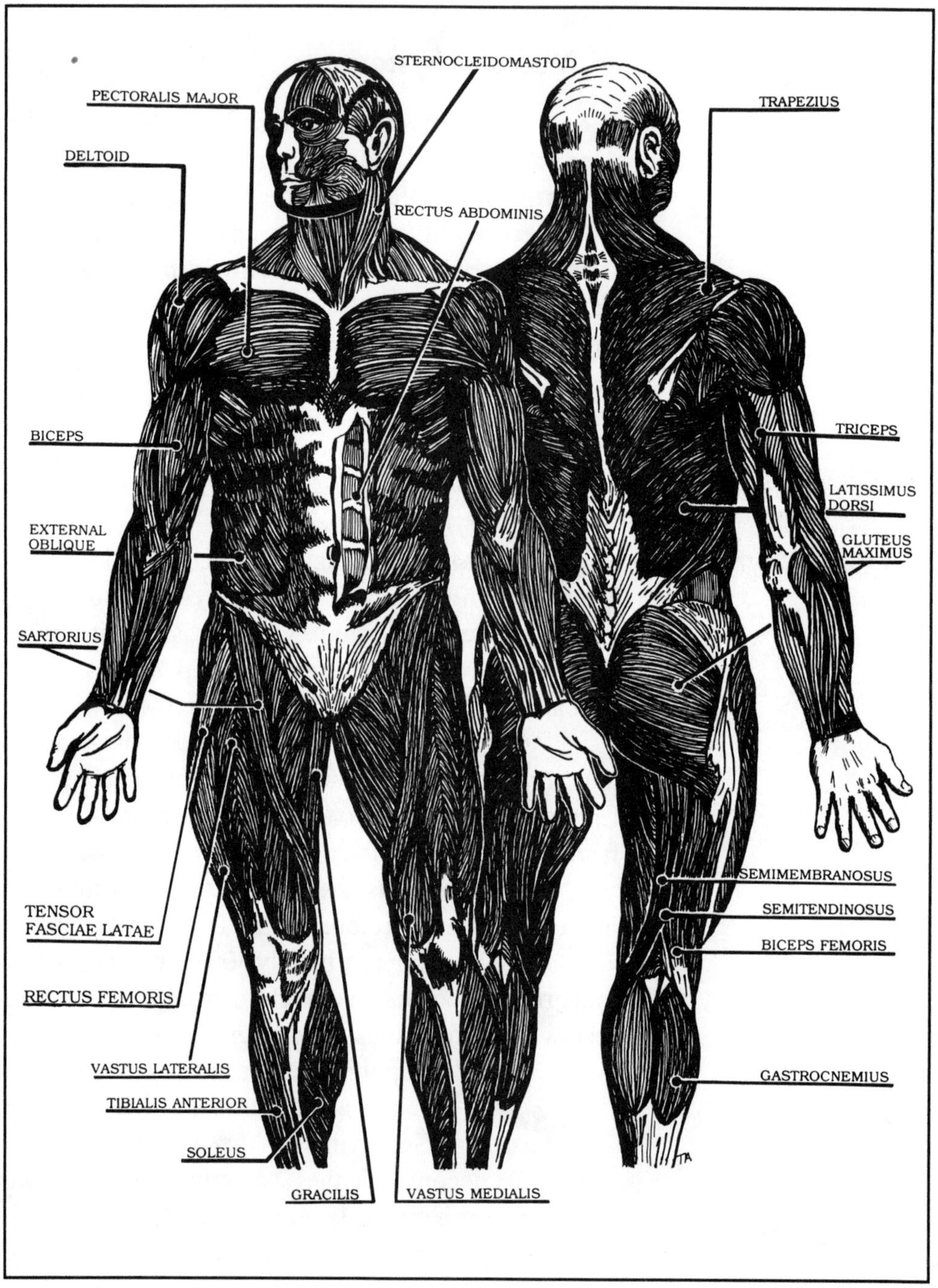

muscle length and consequently a change in segment position. Any active, conscious movement is the result of a change in muscle length. An example is flexing the lower leg at the knee while standing. The hamstring muscle fibers shorten pulling the lower leg toward the buttocks. **Isokinetic** contractions are characterized by movement at a constant velocity. This is only possible using computerized rehabilitation devices.

There are four aspects of muscle function intimately related to Sports Medicine. The first is **flexibility**, which is defined as the range of movement available at a given joint when a body segment is acted on by an internal muscular or external force. Since athletic competition involves various forms of movement at different joint angles, athletes who have greater flexibility will have less chance of injury. In certain activities, a lack of flexibility even causes decreased athletic performance. For these reasons, flexibility training is an important part of every training regime (see Stretching, section 3.1).

Another important aspect of muscle is **strength**, which refers to the amount of force generated by muscle tissue. An increase in force is generated by an increase in the *size* of the muscle fibers, *not* by increasing the number of muscle fibers. This increase in muscle fiber size is called **hypertrophy**, which is seen in weight lifters when their muscles increase in size because of resistance training.

Strength is closely related to **power**, which is defined as strength per unit of time. So, if one athlete can lift a certain amount of weight in half the time another athlete takes, he would have twice the power.

The last aspect, but probably the most important from a coaching perspective, is **muscular endurance**, or the degree to which muscle tissue can maintain contractions against a given force. The limiting factor of this endurance is usually the cardiorespiratory system, which is responsible for transporting oxygen to the muscle cells. The extent to which this system delivers oxygen is referred to as **cardiorespiratory endurance**. If the muscle cells use more oxygen than is delivered by the blood, they suffer **oxygen debt**. These oxygen-deprived cells become less efficient and produce **lactic acid**, which causes muscle soreness. This subject will be examined in detail in section 2.2, Cardiovascular Conditioning.

All muscles that produce movement cross at least one articulation, or joint. Most muscles are connected to bone by **tendons**, although some muscle fibers attach directly to bone, usually forming a broad attachment that allows greater multi-directional movement.

Anatomically, skeletal muscles have at least two attachments: an **origin** and an **insertion**. The origin is attached on the more stable bone, while the insertion is usually tendinous and attached to the more moveable bone. For example, the bicep has two main attachments: the forearm and upper arm. When the bicep is flexed, the forearm attachment moves much more (insertion) than the upper arm attachment (origin).

Muscles are grouped in pairs that function in two ways. If the muscles perform opposite **flexion/extension** functions, such as biceps and triceps, then one group must contract while the other relaxes (figure 1-11). This is the **agonist/antagonist** relationship. The agonists, or movers, are muscles that cause, or help cause a movement. For instance, the biceps in the previous example are the agonists. To facilitate movement, the antagonists, or opposite group, must fully relax to allow proper range of motion.

Muscles may be grouped so that they work together to produce the same movement. Since adjacent muscles pull from the same direction, their respective forces are additive, allowing a more powerful movement. This group effort of certain muscles, which is seen in the four quadricep muscles, is called **synergy** (figure 1-12).

figures 1-11 & 1-12. (Left) Muscle grouping showing the agonist/antagonist relationship. Antagonist must fully relax during agonist contraction to allow a full range of movement. (Right) A synergistic grouping of muscles provides greater strength potential because muscles are working to produce the same movement.

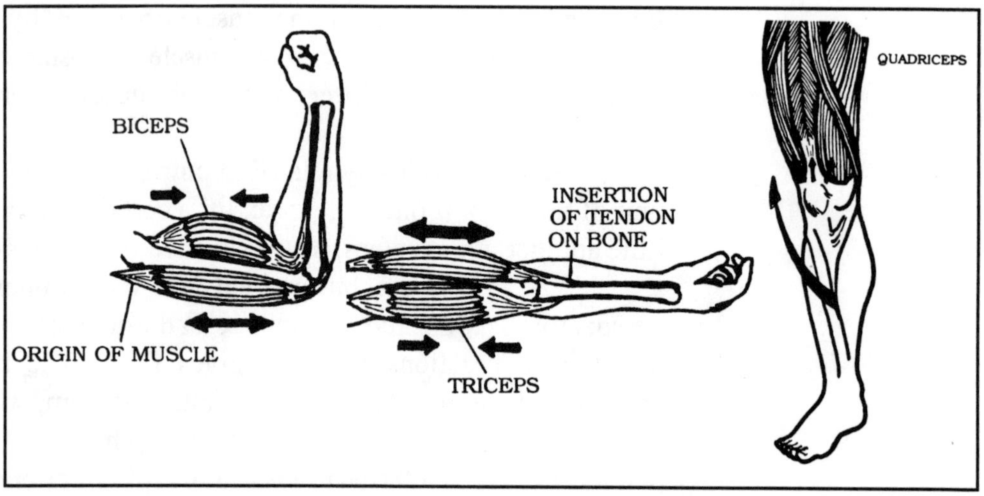

Muscle contraction is very complex. If you would like to know more, you may want to read some texts on human physiology. There are, however, certain fundamental aspects of muscle contraction all coaches should understand.

Muscle fibers are composed of two main proteins: **actin** and **myosin**. During nervous stimulation of a muscle, **calcium** is released, which allows myosin to bind to actin. Myosin creates a ratchet-like force that allows actin to slide by the myosin, causing contraction.

The terminal ends of the nerves that **innervate**, or stimulate, the skeletal muscles are called **motor units**. When a motor unit is stimulated, the corresponding muscle cell fully contracts. This property of muscle in which only *full* contraction of a fiber is possible is called the **all or none response**. If an overall increase in muscle force is needed, more motor units must be stimulated, which in turn contracts more muscle fibers. This is called **recruitment**. Frequency and synchronization of the nervous stimulation also affect a muscle's force.

Since muscle contraction is caused by nervous stimulation, the electrical conduction of the signal becomes very important. Certain elements, namely **potassium**, **sodium** and **chloride**, actually conduct electrical impulses and are thus called **electrolytes**. Besides conduction, electrolytes are responsible for maintaining fluid balance in the muscles. A lack of electrolytes, which is normally brought about by excessive fluid loss, can cause cramping and muscle spasms.

Temperature is another factor that affects muscle performance. It has been shown that the **deep muscle**, or **core**, **temperature** is directly related to the speed of contraction and relaxation. In other words, if muscles are warmed up properly, they contract and relax faster, which increases athletic potential. In fact, warm-up exercises like those in section 3.2 raise inner core muscle temperatures much more effectively than external heating by heat packs, etc.

All humans have two main muscle fiber types. **Slow twitch fibers** have a high endurance, or aerobic capacity, but their contraction speed is slower and less forceful than the fast twitch fibers. Conversely, **fast twitch fibers** have a high anaerobic capacity (see section 2.2) and produce a rapid and forceful contraction. Current research indicates that the percentage of the respective fiber types is primarily determined genetically, although fiber composition has been shown to change in athletes who train rigorously.

Muscle metabolism in training is discussed at length in section 2.3. Study figure 1-10 to become familiar with the human body's major muscles, which are key elements in athletic success.

1.3 MOVEMENT AND DIRECTION

The study of human movement is called **kinesiology**. There is a remarkably wide range of movements possible, but there are some general rules that help us better understand movement. These rules, however, must be applied cautiously.

All movements occur around an **axis**, or pivot point, and along a **plane** (figure 1-13). Because the study of axis and planes is complicated, movements are most often characterized by joint angles and positions relative to a standard

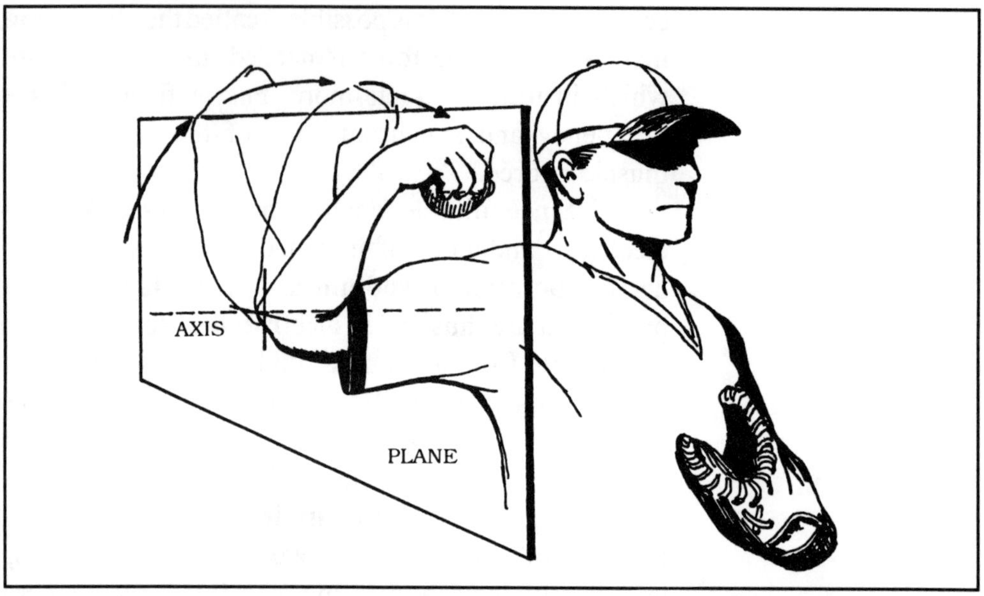

figure 1-13. Movement around an axis and along a plane.

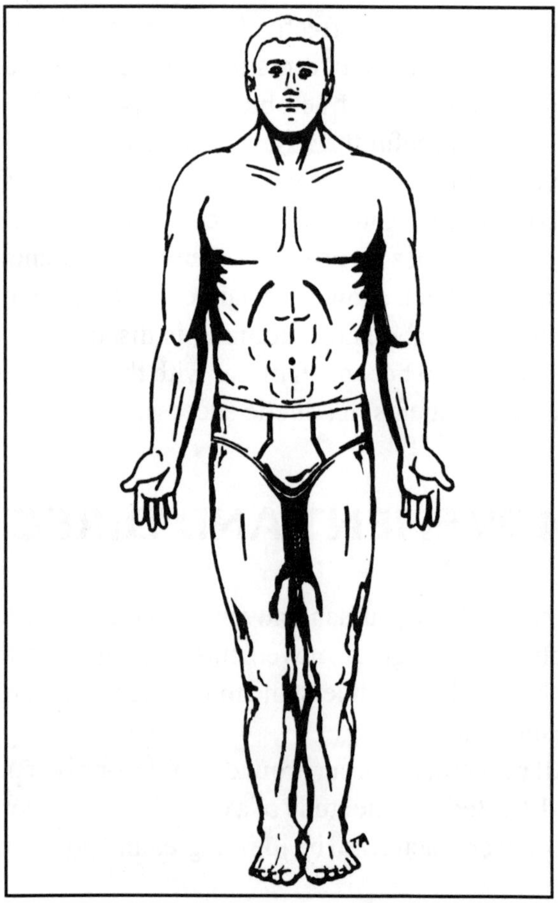

figure 1-14. Anatomical position. Feet are together, and palms are facing forward.

position called the **anatomical position**, in which all joints are extended and palms are facing forward (figure 1-14). From this position, if any body segment is moved, it must be flexion as long as the involved joint's angle is reduced. In other words, turning the head from side to side is not flexion because the involved joint angle is not reduced. On the other hand, if the foot is kicked back toward the buttocks, the knee joint angle is decreased, so the movement is flexion (figure 1-15).

If the joint angle is increased, the movement is called **extension**. If the extension is continued past normal anatomical position, it is referred to as **hyperextension**, which occurs at the wrist joint normally and is seen in many other injuries.

The ankle is a special joint that is capable of a wide variety of movements. Because of this, ankle movements have their own separate terminology. Upward flexion of the ankle is called **dorsiflexion**, and downward extension past neutral position is called **plantarflexion** (figure 1-16). An inward movement of the toes is referred to as **inversion**, and an outward movement is called **eversion**.

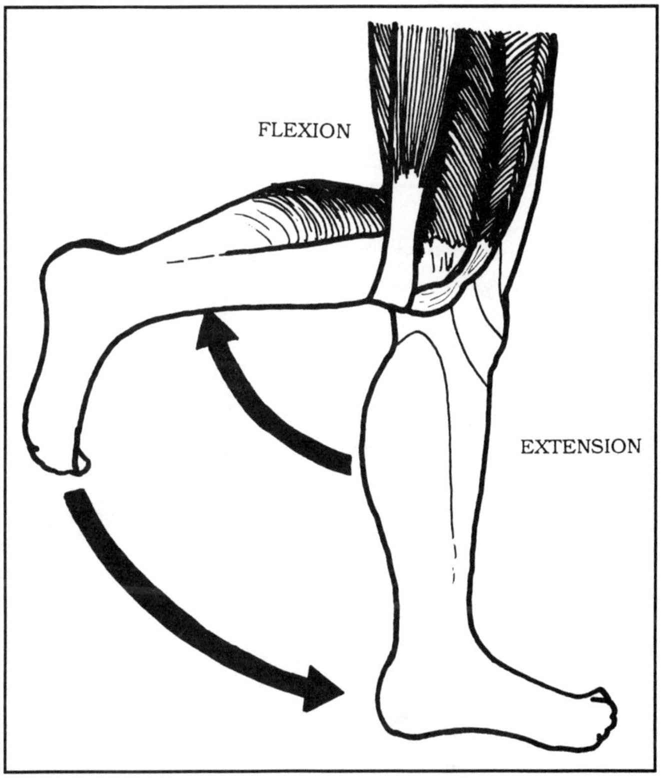

figure 1-15. Flexion and extension of the lower leg.

As you may remember from the glossary in section 1.1, movement away from the midline of the body is **abduction** and movement towards midline is **adduction**. Any circular motion of the shoulder or hip joint is referred to as **circumduction** (figure 1-17).

In addition to understanding movement, coaches must be familiar with body position and direction. This is especially important when communicating with medical professionals. A body part closer to the midline is referred to as **medial**. A part farther from the midline is called **lateral** (figure 1-18). Body parts can also be described by their position relative to the heart. A body part that is closer to the heart is **proximal**, while a more distant part is **distal**. For example, the inner part of the knee is medial compared to the lateral outside of the joint. The knee would be proximal to the ankle.

Structures may also be named according to their position relative to the top of the head. If one part is, anatomically speaking, closer to the head than another part, it is **superior**. The lower part is called **inferior**. In cases of long structures such as the vena cava vein, the upper portion is called the superior vena cava to indicate that a lower region exists.

figure 1-16. Ankle movements.

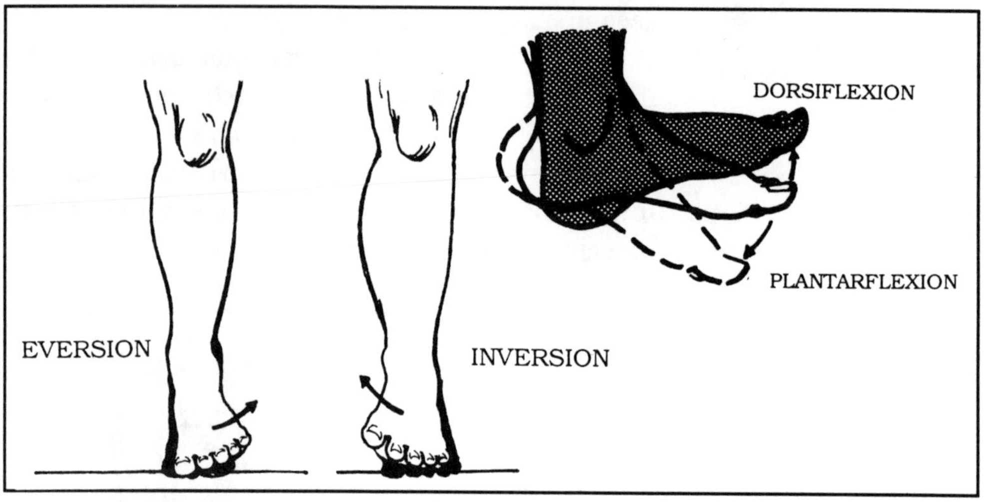

In addition to position and movement relative to other body parts, joint motion can be described by the *amount* of movement. The total amount of movement possible at a certain joint is its **range of motion (ROM)**. Two terms used synonymously with ROM are **mobility** and **flexibility**. ROM is determined largely by the shape of the articulating bones and the tightness of the surrounding ligament and muscle tissue. Thus, stretching is extremely important in increasing flexibility. Flexible joints are just as strong as inflexible joints, but the increased ROM allows a flexible articulation to move safely into positions that an inflexible one cannot assume. This is why flexibility is one of the most important parts of injury prevention.

figure 1-17. Various movements of the arms. It is easy to remember ADDuction is ADDing a body part, or moving it toward the body. CIRCumduction is a CIRCular movement.

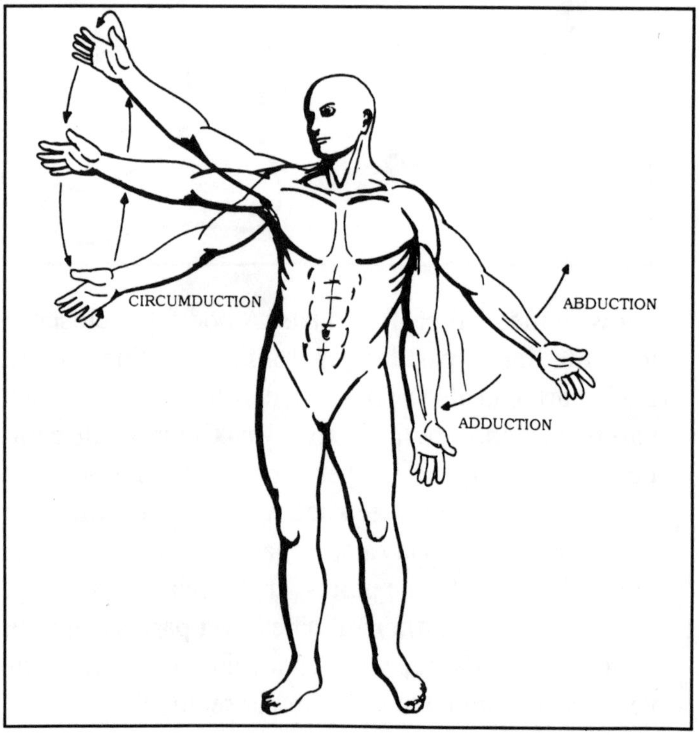

Another concept useful in understanding movement is **center of gravity (COG)**. Every object on the figure 1-18. Positional relationships of the knee and ankle. Knee (A) is superior and proximal to the ankle (B). The medial side of the knee is closest to the midline of the body.

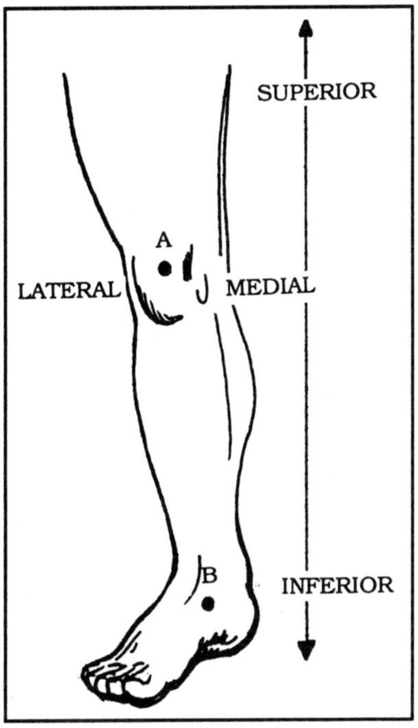

earth's surface is subject to the force of gravity. If you imagine that this force is concentrated at a single point in the body, it would be the body's center of gravity. In other words, the COG is the point where the body's weight is concentrated. Closely related to COG is the **base of support (BOS)**, which is the area bounded by the body parts in contact with the ground (figure 1-19). **Balance** is defined as the state in which a body's COG passes through some part of its BOS. From these definitions it is easy to see why we are more stable standing on two feet than on one: Our base of support is larger, and therefore it is easier to keep the COG within the boundaries of the BOS to maintain balance.

figure 1-19. Athlete on left is balanced because his center of gravity (COG) passes through his base of support (BOS). Athlete on right is unbalanced because his BOS is cut in half and, consequently, his COG falls outside his support.

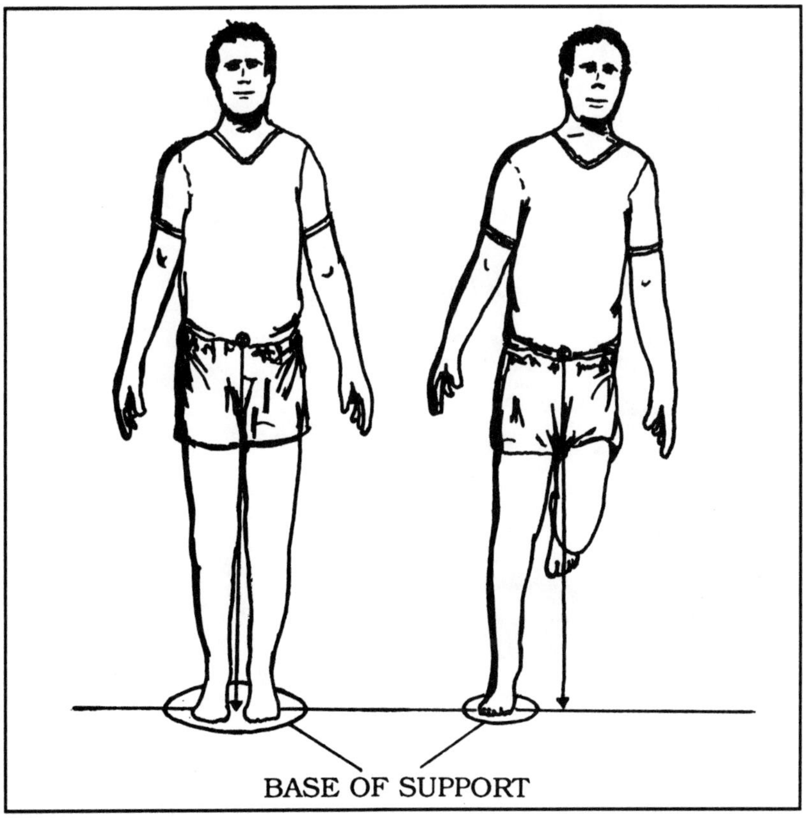

The COG varies more laterally as the distance from the COG to the ground increases. Since COG must be kept within the BOS, a lower COG will increase the **stability** of a body.

The basic terminology, systems and principles discussed in Chapter 1 should help any coach or athlete better understand how the body works and how to keep it at its peak.

2 Athletic Health and Fitness

People are more health and fitness conscious today than perhaps any other previous generation. Despite this heightened awareness, non-athletes have much different needs than those people who train to compete in athletic events.

This chapter, which covers wellness, conditioning and weight control, is devoted to the health, fitness and therefore happiness of all athletes.

2.1 GENERAL BODY WELLNESS

Daily body maintenance is important for everybody, but especially for athletes who strive for maximal performance. Athletes need to consider these six components of wellness:

- •Proper sleep
- •Mental health
- •Personal hygiene
- •No misuse of drugs and alcohol
- •Plenty of exercise
- •Proper nutrition.

SLEEP

Most professionals agree that the majority of athletes need a minimum seven hours of sleep each night. Normal sleep habits, however, vary widely, so athletes should continue their present sleep routine if it makes them feel sufficiently rested.

Sleep rests the mind, not just the body, which makes proper sleep necessary every night, not just before or after competition. Many athletes feel anxious and sleep fitfully the night before an event, so it is especially important that they get a good night's sleep two nights before competition to ensure their minds are as relaxed as possible.

MENTAL HEALTH

In this context, mental health refers to internal happiness. Athletes should be satisfied with themselves and their performances. They should be encouraged to achieve, but should not push beyond normal limits. Any negative stress such as mental manipulation, excessive anxiety, overtraining or verbal degradation can lead to decreased psychological wellness. Chapter 4 talks more about coaching techniques to encourage top performance.

DRUGS AND ALCOHOL

Drugs and alcohol decrease performance as well as consistency. Many drugs, such as alcohol, have substantial detrimental effects for athletes, including impaired reaction, diuresis (excessive fluid loss in the form of urine) and deep sleep inhibition. Athletes should certainly avoid all "social" drugs, especially during the competitive season. Drugs add stress to an already stressed body and actually diminish athletic performance. If you would like more information, consult texts on drugs and alcohol in athletics.

EXERCISE

Exercise has many positive effects on the body, yet at the same time it also stresses the body. For this reason, this sort of stress is called **positive stress.**

All individuals should exercise because, among other attributes, it:

- •Decreases probability of cardiovascular disease
- •Decreases cancer potential
- •Increases quality of sleep
- •Increases mental health
- •Increases cardiovascular and respiratory efficiency.

ATHLETIC NUTRITION

Athletes, coaches and Sports Medicine specialists all recognize the importance of sports nutrition. There is no doubt that a balanced diet—which requires eating the right foods at the right times—substantially benefits athletes and their performances.

After all, exercise makes demands on all systems of the body. For proper maintenance, recovery and repair of these systems, a balanced diet is essential.

At the amateur level, athletes and their parents often rely on the coaches for nutritional guidance.

Basic Nutrition

Foods can be divided into six basic groups:

- Carbohydrates
- Proteins
- Fats
- Water
- Vitamins
- Minerals.

Carbohydrates are the body's first choice for fuel. They are easily broken down and, when metabolized, produce water and carbon dioxide that can be eliminated through sweating and breathing. Carbohydrates are divided into two groups: simple and complex. **Simple** carbohydrates are found in foods sweetened with sugars, either sucrose (table sugar) or fructose (sugar in fruit). These sugars are absorbed quickly into the blood stream providing a fast, short-term energy boost. **Complex** carbohydrates are found in foods containing starch such as pastas and potatoes. These carbohydrates are absorbed slower and provide a gradual energy increase, and are therefore recommended while training. All carbohydrates prevent gastric stress during digestion because they break down so easily.

The body uses **proteins** primarily for growth and maintenance. Protein is the body's last choice for energy because it is difficult to break down. Proteins are divided into two forms: complete and incomplete. **Complete** proteins are found in milk, meat, eggs, fish, etc. They contain all the essential **amino acids**, or protein sub-units, that cannot be synthesized by the body. **Incomplete proteins** are found in cereals and vegetables. They do not contain all the essential amino acids, which is why vegetarians must have a knowledge of which vegetables have the necessary proteins to ensure a balanced diet.

Fat is a backup source of energy. It is also the only substance the body continues to store beyond required amounts, which is why some people become overweight. Fats, also, are divided into two groups: saturated and unsaturated. **Saturated fats** are found in meats, eggs, milk, etc., while **unsaturated fats** are found in vegetables. The body has more difficulty breaking down the saturated fats. Experts say 30% of your diet should consist of fat calories, which is quite easy with the typical American diet!

Water comprises about 71% of our body's volume and is used in every body process. Everyone should consume at least four tall glasses of water each day and increase the amount according to the level of activity and amount of sweat lost. Because of their high level of activity, athletes and coaches must constantly guard against dehydration. Studies now indicate that drinking small, frequent amounts of water is better for maintaining fluid levels during hot weather and strenuous competition.

Vitamins promote good health, prevent deficiency diseases and regulate body processes. Although vitamins are not a source of energy, they are important for normal body function and should be replaced every day.

The body, however, is capable of producing only three vitamins: A, D and K. The other needed vitamins are E, B_1 (thiamin), B_2 (riboflavin), B_3 (niacin), B_6, folic acid, B_{12}, biotin, pantothenic acid and C (ascorbic acid). If an athlete eats healthy, well-balanced meals, there is usually no need for vitamin supplements.

Minerals augment the body processes and help them run smoothly. The body also requires twelve minerals each day; most important are calcium, iodine, iron, sodium, chloride and potassium. The latter three minerals are needed for

table 2-1. Daily dietary requirements from the four food groups.

FOOD GROUP	NUMBER OF DAILY SERVINGS	EXAMPLES OF FOODS
MILK	2/ADULTS 3/CHILDREN 4/TEENAGERS	LOW-FAT MILK, COTTAGE CHEESE, ICE CREAM, YOGURT, CHEESE
MEAT	2	RED MEAT, DRY BEANS, PEAS, NUTS, FISH, POULTRY, EGGS
FRUIT AND VEGETABLES	4	DARK GREEN OR ORANGE VEGETABLES, CITRUS FRUIT
BREAD AND CEREAL	4	BREAD, CEREAL, RICE, OATS, PASTA

fluid balance, muscle activity and cell metabolism. A balanced diet usually supplies all necessary minerals.

No single food contains all the essential vitamins, minerals and sources of energy (protein, fat, and carbohydrates) in the amounts the body needs. Part of a balanced diet is selecting a variety of foods from each of the four basic food groups.

Nutritional Content of Food Groups

MILK PRODUCTS

Milk is high in protein, calcium, phosphorus, niacin, riboflavin and vitamins A and D. Try lower-in-fat milk products. If you are drinking whole milk, which is 4% fat, try 2% fat milk. Also, look for milk products fortified with vitamins A and D. It is important to note that there is no nutritional difference between whole and skim milk, besides fat. Adults and young children need two servings daily; older children, teenagers and pregnant or breast-feeding women need three to four servings.

MEAT, POULTRY, SEAFOOD, NUTS, EGGS, DRIED BEANS AND PEAS

These foods are high in protein, B vitamins, iron and other minerals. Trim the skin off chicken and turkey, and trim all visible fat off lean beef, veal, pork and lamb. Rabbit, pheasant, venison, wild duck and other wild game generally have less fat than domestically raised animals. All types of fish and shellfish are good, although you should limit consumption of shrimp, lobster and sardines to *no more than* one serving per week. A few times a week, try "low-meat" or "no-meat" recipes that include dried beans, peas, lentils, soybean curd (tofu), peanut butter or low-fat cheese. Also try combining small amounts of meat, fish or poultry with rice or pasta in mixed dishes or casseroles.

Adults need no more than two small servings (about five to seven ounces) of meat, poultry or seafood daily. A three-ounce portion might contain:

- Half a chicken breast or a chicken leg and a thigh
- A half-cup of flaked fish
- Two thin slices lean roast beef.

Preschool children should have about one ounce of meat, poultry or seafood per day for each year of age.

FRUITS AND VEGETABLES

Fruits and vegetables are high in vitamins, minerals, potassium and fiber, and low in fat, calories and sodium. They contain *no* cholesterol. Asparagus, broccoli, cabbage, cantaloupe, grapefruit, greens (mustard, beet, kale, collards), green pepper, oranges, potatoes, spinach, strawberries, tangerines and tomatoes are high in vitamin C. Broccoli, cantaloupe, carrots, greens, peaches, pumpkin, spinach, sweet potatoes and winter squash are high in vitamin A.

Enjoy plenty of vegetables and fruits. If you are watching your weight, these foods will give you the most nutrition for the fewest calories.

BREADS, CEREALS, PASTA AND STARCHY VEGETABLES

These foods are high in B vitamins, iron and fiber, and low in fat and cholesterol. All kinds of breads (wheat, rye, raisin, white) are good; those with whole-grain or enriched flours are best. All types of hot and cold vegetables, rices and pastas made without egg are good additions to your diet. Potatoes, lima beans, green peas, winter squash, corn, yams or sweet potatoes are starchy vegetables that help balance your diet.

Athletic Nutrition No-No's

Although good nutrition is important for everyone, *athletes have special needs*. Some things to avoid are:

- Drinking coffee, colas and other caffeine-laden substances on the day of competition.

Caffeine stimulates the brain and adrenal system. The body, however, has a limited amount of adrenalin stored in the adrenal glands. When caffeine enters the bloodstream, adrenalin is released, which adds pep. But when caffeine is consumed before rigorous competition, the body's reserves of adrenalin are partially used up, leaving minimal adrenalin for competition. In addition, many caffeinated beverages cause fluid loss.

- Drinking heavily sweetened drinks during competition, especially sodas, Kool-Aid™, sweet lemonade, Gatorade™, etc.

Sugar slows the absorption of fluids from the stomach to the body systems. Sugar also produces a feeling of fullness and thus further limits water intake. High sugar drinks should generally be given *after*, not during games.

Electrolyte drinks such as Gatorade™, Power Burst™, etc. should be diluted with four parts water to one part electrolyte drink if they are going to be ingested during competition.

•Eating steak and eggs before competition.

Complex proteins take five to six hours to leave the stomach area. Excessive amounts of food in the stomach during competition can lead to cramps, excess stomach acid and diaphragm restriction, which affects breathing. Also, protein wastes can only be eliminated through urine, which increases urinary system stress.

Pre-Activity Nutrition

Thorough research indicates that dietary habits significantly influence pre-activity stress factors such as stomach cramps, excess stomach acid, dry mouth and dizziness.

Athletes' pre-competition meals should suite their tastes as well as assure them that the food will contribute to performance. Of course, pre-activity meals cannot supply all the energy athletes need for events. In fact, the foods eaten during the other days of the week supply most of the required energy. That's why some athletes who get highly emotional before competition find it counterproductive to eat before an event, but can still compete.

Pre-activity meals should be eaten two-and-a-half to three hours before competition and ideally should be:

•Low in fats (salads and breads)
•Low in proteins (pastas)
•Low in spices (macaroni and cheese)
•High in carbohydrates and sugars (peanut butter and jelly sandwiches, granola)
•Easily absorbable by the body (crackers, liquid food supplements).

Eating these foods decreases the time it takes to process them, turn them into fuel and clear the stomach area. Commercial food supplements are often beneficial during pre-competition meals because of their high calorie content, low metabolism time and wide range of vitamins and minerals. A good pre-activity meal might be spaghetti with tomato sauce, French bread, tossed salad with Italian dressing, fresh fruit and water.

For activities that require long-term endurance, such as marathons and triathalons, most athletes start their nutritional preparation 48 hours before the start of competition by consuming a well-balanced diet high in carbohydrates.

A rather new and still unproven approach is "carbohydrate loading" or "charging." Athletes drain their body's supplies of glycogen in the muscles and liver four to six days before the event by eating foods low in carbohydrates. Then, three days prior to competition, they "load" their bodies with "carbos" in hopes of supercharging their body reserves of glycogen for competition.

It is the coach's and athlete's responsibility to follow proper pre-activity nutrition.

2.2 CARDIOVASCULAR CONDITIONING

Athletes' bodies must be prepared for the stresses they must withstand during competition, and that preparation should begin four to six weeks before the event. Athletes are constantly subjected to two kinds of stress: positive stress, which is created by exercise, and **negative stress**, which is caused by anxiety, illness, an unbalanced diet or injury. Positive stress is good for the body and should be encouraged, while negative stress should be avoided as much as possible.

Training programs are designed to increase flexibility (section 3.1), coordination and agility (section 3.4) and conditioning, which is the focus of this section. Since some athletic events require long, sustained effort, while others require short bursts of energy, coaches must be careful to adhere to training principles that increase fitness for each specific sport or event.

AEROBIC CONDITIONING

To condition for endurance, an athlete wants to increase the efficiency with which the body delivers oxygen to the tissues. If more oxygen is delivered, the cells can continue to efficiently make energy from food. This process of increasing oxygen uptake is called **aerobic conditioning**. To fully understand this concept, we must first look at some basics.

Three forms of food are used as energy:

- •Carbohydrates
- •Fats
- •Proteins.

These three differ in their energy efficiency and ease of use. The body's first choice for fuel is carbohydrates, followed by fat and, finally, protein. This is because carbohydrates use less oxygen to burn the same amount of energy and are therefore more efficient.

The body has two pathways to produce energy. If there is adequate oxygen present in the blood, nutrient molecules will follow the oxidative pathway, which is a relatively efficient system. A large amount of energy molecules (adenosine triphosphate, or ATP) are produced while carbon dioxide (CO_2) and water are produced as waste products. This is beneficial because CO_2 is easily removed by the cardiorespiratory system, and water is needed by the body. Therefore, the oxidative, or **aerobic**, pathway does not tax other body systems by producing harmful by-products.

The second energy pathway is **anaerobic respiration**. This occurs when the cardiorespiratory system cannot meet the needs of the respiring cells and, as a result, must produce energy in the *absence* of oxygen. This process is relatively *inefficient* because only a few ATP energy molecules are produced. Meanwhile, lactic acid is being produced as a by-product. **Lactic acid** is a toxic substance that causes muscle soreness and must be converted into a non-toxic compound as soon as oxygen is available. Lactic acid also is an acidic molecule and consequently decreases the pH of the blood. This drastically affects other body systems, allowing the body to function normally only for short periods once lactic acid is present in the blood.

Since a buildup of lactic acid quickly decreases the body's ability to function, athletes in long distance events actively avoid it. In other words, they use the aerobic pathway and, as they train, make many important body adjustments to prevent the lactic acid buildup created by anaerobic respiration. Athletes become more efficient at delivering oxygen to their cells by increasing the amount of capillaries in their muscle tissue, increasing the efficiency of their heart contractions, increasing the ability of the blood and muscles to uptake oxygen, and increasing the efficiency of the pulmonary system (lungs). Besides these changes, the body will store more glycogen (complex units of glucose) molecules in the muscle tissue to increase energy storage, and will also produce blood buffers that prevent the blood pH from dropping, or becoming acidic, if some lactic acid is present. Obviously, aerobic conditioning drastically changes the internal chemistry of the body, making it a much more efficient energy-producing machine.

Since the cardiorespiratory system is the limiting factor in aerobic conditioning, **heart rate** is a good indicator of the exercise stress level. If the heart is beating fast, the cells must be using more oxygen, which forces the heart to rush oxygenated blood to the tissues. The heart can only beat at a certain pace, however, which in referred to as the maximum heart rate (MAX HR). MAX HR decreases proportionally with age.

Aerobic conditioning is defined as exercising continually at 65-80% of MAX HR for at least 20 minutes. You can determine MAX HR by using this equation:

MAX HR = 220 - [YOUR AGE] **(1)**

To determine your aerobic target zone, use this equation:

UPPER AEROBIC ZONE=MAX HR x .8
LOWER AEROBIC ZONE=MAX HR x .65 **(2)**

This information can also be found in table 2-2.

table 2.2. Aerobic and advanced conditioning pulse rate zones. Pulse rate is equal to the number of heart beats per minute (see figure 2-1).

AGE	HR MAX	65-80% AEROBIC ZONE	85% ZONE FOR CONDITIONED ATHLETES
10	210	137-168	179
15	205	133-164	174
20	200	130-160	170
25	195	127-156	166
30	190	124-152	162
35	185	120-148	157
40	180	117-144	153
45	175	114-140	149
50	170	111-136	145
55	165	107-132	140

These values are general and fit about 90% of the population. About 10% of the population, however, has either enlarged or extremely small hearts, which changes the maximum heart rate values and consequently the aerobic zone. For this reason, it is best to use equation 3 to determine your training zone.

$$\textbf{UPPER TRAINING ZONE} = HR_R + .65(\text{MAX HR} - HR_R)$$
$$\textbf{LOWER TRAINING ZONE} = HR_R + .8(\text{MAX HR} - HR_R) \quad (3)$$

The above equation can be rearranged to find your training intensity (in percent of MAX HR).

$$\%\ \text{MAX HR} = \frac{TZ - HR_R}{\text{MAX HR} - HR_R} \quad (4)$$

TZ -Training zone measured during exercise
HR_R -Resting heart rate
MAX HR -Found using equation (1)

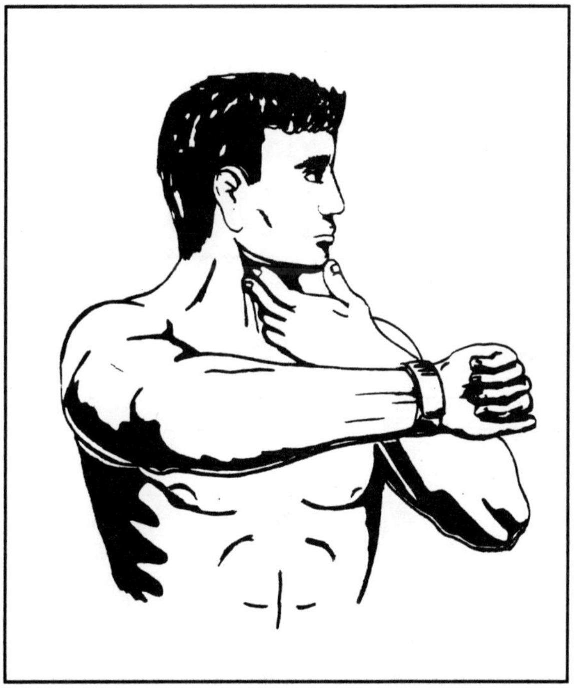

figure 2-1. The carotid pulse can usually be found easier than the wrist pulse during exercise. It is a good idea to practice taking your pulse before exercise begins.

You can monitor your heart rate by taking your pulse, which indicates the number of beats per minute. You'll find the pulse in the neck immediately adjacent to the larynx, where the carotid artery supplies blood to the brain.

When exercising, estimate your pulse rate by:

\# OF BEATS IN 10 SECONDS x 6 = **APPROXIMATE PULSE RATE**

Tips for Aerobic Exercise

To maximize value from aerobic exercise, keep these guidelines in mind:

- Aerobic exercise requires non-stop activity within the training zone for 20 minutes. This does *not* include warm-up time outside the training zone.
- Athletes should train aerobically at least four times a week.
- Maintain a comfortable pace that makes you only slightly winded.
- You must use your legs, but also try to include as many muscle groups as possible.
- Do not compare yourself with others or train with people who are at a different fitness level.

There are many popular aerobic exercises that are easy to integrate into a team or personal program. Table 2-3 includes the approximate time needed to complete your warm-up as well as the required aerobic time.

table 2-3. Aerobic exercises with work out times that fulfill warm-up and aerobic conditioning.

TEAM EXERCISES	WORK OUT TIME	PERSONAL EXERCISES	WORK OUT TIME
Running	20 min	All team exercises	Varies
Jogging	20 min	Cycling	20 min
Aerobic/step classes	40 min	Stair climbing	20 min
Jumping rope	20 min	Cross country skiing	20 min
Swimming	30 min	Rowing	20 min

To avoid boredom, burnout and exercising only a certain group of muscles (and consequently becoming conditioned in only one exercise), athletes should use at least two different exercises in their aerobic training program.

You can evaluate aerobic fitness by various techniques, including:

- Measuring VO_2 MAX (maximum oxygen uptake) in a laboratory
- Noting a decrease in resting pulse rate

- Measuring the time it takes to run a set distance, such as a half-mile or mile. Lower times indicate increased fitness
- Measuring recovery time after running, walking, etc. a set distance, which is normally done by measuring pulse after exercise and recording time until resting pulse value is achieved.

ANAEROBIC CONDITIONING

If an exercise activity is intense, cells require more oxygen than can be delivered by the cardiorespiratory system, which, as we have already discussed, produces lactic acid that then accumulates in the blood. This shortens exercising endurance.

Therefore, anaerobic activities must be short, intense activities, such as:

- Sprinting
- Weight lifting
- Football.

Conditioning for these activities includes increasing the supply of ATP energy molecules stored in the muscle tissue and increasing the blood buffers to help delay the effects of lactic acid production.

TRAINING TECHNIQUES

There is a definite art to conditioning. That art is knowing when more is needed and when enough is enough. Athletes should not be pushed too hard or too fast to avoid both physical and psychological damage.

Conditioning training should start *at least* four weeks before the season begins to ensure the body is ready to compete. Athletes usually begin their program by running until slightly winded, then increase the workout a little each day. They should *not* push as hard when it is hot, and should be constantly monitored for signs of heat exhaustion. *More players die each year from heat-related sickness than any other injury.* Also, athletes who are recovering from illness or injury should ease workouts to facilitate the healing process.

One of the best methods of increasing aerobic and anaerobic fitness simultaneously is to *mix* jogging and wind sprints. Jogging, which is purely aerobic, is combined with sprinting, which is exclusively anaerobic. The method is based on the reasoning that the cardiovascular system is already taxed at 65-80% of its MAX HR, and then it is forced to recover from intense exercise that creates oxygen debt. In other words, your body is forced to recover from a stress (sprinting) when it is already stressed (jogging). Again, athletes should begin such methods *slowly* to avoid negative stresses on the body.

Remember, the goal of conditioning is to ensure athletic preservation, so good judgment is an important aspect of every conditioning program.

2.3 DIETING AND WEIGHT LOSS

An athlete's body is a finely-tuned machine. All negative stresses—including a poor or insufficient diet—will have a marked detrimental effect on performance. This is why most competitive athletes are discouraged from dieting. From a realistic point of view, however, athletes can perform better when they are at an ideal weight for their body type. There are proven weight-loss techniques that do not involve what we normally think of as "dieting" that we will discuss shortly.

First, though, we must distinguish between **overweight** and **overfat**. Certain tables provide an ideal weight for a certain height. Although these may be of value to the general public, they are not appropriate for athletes whose bodies often are heavy for their height because of muscle mass. This muscle, called **lean body mass (LBM)**, is actually beneficial for most athletic activities. With this in mind, athletes should never sacrifice muscle mass and should lose weight only if they are overfat.

Total body weight is equal to LBM plus the weight of fat. This fat mass should be the target of any weight-loss program. Normal fat values are different for men and women. Because their bodies require fat for certain feminine body processes, women normally have at least 10% more fat than men. Normal values for different groups are shown below.

Before beginning a weight-loss program, an athlete must determine that he or she is overfat. This can be accomplished by **hydrostatic**, or underwater, weighing or by **anthropometric measurement**, for which a qualified technician uses skin calipers.

If an athlete wants to lose fat, the decision requires real commitment.

Since dieting techniques can be harmful to athletic performance, athletes must lose weight by changing their lifestyle. An athlete must drop 3,500 calories under normal body needs to lose one pound of fat. From this we can see that the "miracle" diets that supposedly enable dieters to lose two to five pounds per week are actually causing the loss of something other than fat (which just happens to be water). Consider, too, that normal caloric intake is between 1,500 and 3,000 calories per day. If one pound of fat is lost in a week (a 3,500 calorie deficit), then the body is deprived of 500 calories a day, which is approximately a 15% drop. This suggests the diet is probably not well-balanced or nutritionally sound, especially for athletes.

table 2-4. Fat percentage classifications.

	NORMAL FAT %	OVER FAT %	IDEAL ATHLETIC FAT %	NECESSARY FAT %
WOMEN	19-25	>25	10-19	10
MEN	12-18	>18	3-14	3

Since a large reduction in caloric intake is not wise, we can look to exercise for a possible calorie-burning solution. Twenty minutes of jogging, however, only burns 180 calories, a little more than two pieces of plain whole wheat bread. It should be obvious that exercise itself cannot burn enough calories to lose weight.

The answer lies in the **basal metabolic rate (BMR)** that, as you remember, is the rate at which cells burn calories while the body is at rest. Regular participation in an aerobic exercise program of at least 20 to 30 minutes of continuous exercise, four days a week, usually increases the BMR. Since 90% of the body's energy is used in muscle metabolism, an increased BMR offers major fat-burning potential. This change allows more energy (fat) to be burnt as heat instead of being stored, promotes changes in blood pH to decrease hunger, and increases muscle enzymes while decreasing fat-storing enzymes. This process involves a gradual change of internal chemistry, and noticeable results are sometimes not observed for six months.

When muscles are exercised, they normally use about 60 to 70% fat and 30 to 40% carbohydrates. As the exercise intensity increases, the body switches to larger and larger percentages of carbohydrates until it reaches 100% carbohydrate metabolism. This is because fat takes more oxygen to table 2-5. Ideal exercise intensities for burning fat.

AGE	HR MAX	65-70% FAT BURNING ZONE
10	210	137-147
15	205	133-144
20	200	130-140
25	195	127-137
30	190	124-133
35	185	120-130
40	180	117-126
45	175	114-123
50	170	111-119
55	165	107-116

burn. If there is a shortage of oxygen in the blood (intense exercise), the body cannot spare oxygen to burn fat, and consequently burns only carbohydrates. The ideal fat burning intensity is therefore 65 to 70% MAX HR. Pulse values are available in table 2-5.

Since fat burning requires low to moderate intensity, athletes should exercise *longer*, not harder. The key factor seems to be the amount of time spent at 65 to 70% MAX HR, which not only burns the highest fat percentages, but also induces the largest amount of metabolic change.

Prolonged exercise also stimulates DNA (which carries the genetic information in the cell) to produce fat-burning enzymes that allow a greater percentage of fat metabolism.

The second part of this fat-loss technique consists of changing eating habits. First, fat intake must be decreased. The recommended daily fat intake is 30% of the ingested calories. If, however, an athlete wishes to lose fat at a reasonably rapid rate, this percentage should be close to 20, with approximately 7% from monounsaturated, 7% from polyunsaturated and 7% from saturated fats. Be sure to consult a dietician for proper guidance of caloric intake and the nutritional value of foods.

Second, the diet should be well-balanced. Meals should consist of selections from each of the four food groups (p. 52-54). With the exception of fat intake, the diet should consist of everyday foods, just in smaller portions. It is important, especially during training, to eat adequate protein and carbohydrates to ensure proper body maintenance. Athletes should *never* starve themselves by severely cutting caloric intake, because it can trigger undesirable effects such as muscle loss, decreased athletic performance and possibly create a **craving-binging cycle**.

These cycles are typically seen in individuals who are anxious about their caloric intake. Consequently, they avoid foods they enjoy because of their high fat content. After about a week of this denial, their craving for a specific food becomes so great that they binge, or eat the food in excessive amounts. This normal psychological occurrence means that athletes *will* eat foods they enjoy, regardless of good intentions. So it is critical not to remove certain enjoyable foods such as chocolate and other sweets from the diet. The trick is to consume very small amounts of these enjoyable foods every day. In a matter of weeks, these foods will become routine and monotonous, and the cycle will be broken. Athletes must not, however, misinterpret this information to mean they should stuff themselves with fattening foods to avoid craving. Instead, if athletes suffer from craving, they must pick one favorite food and eat very small amounts daily.

So, if an athlete wants to lose fat, the BMR must be increased by aerobic exercise using the largest amount of muscle groups possible. The amount of exercise at 65 to 70% MAX HR seems to be directly proportional to the amount of metabolic change toward increased fat-burning efficiency. At the same time, the diet should be well-balanced but portions should be smaller. Athletes should avoid large meals and craving of certain foods.

Lastly, do not look to the scale for results. It does not indicate metabolic change; only fat testing shows the real improvement.

DIETING FACTS

Coaches and athletes should keep these facts about dieting in mind:

- Dieting is not an effective weight-loss method for athletes.

Strict dieting forces the body to lose water and **subcutaneous fat,** which is the fat below the skin. These diets do not, however, affect the amount of intramuscular fat and do not change the level of fat-burning or fat-storing enzymes. Therefore, the metabolism is not changed, and the dieter must continually diet or the weight will be regained immediately. Also, since intramuscular fat levels are unchanged, body composition tests show little fat percentage change even though weight is lost.

- Fasting or low-calorie diets increase fat weight.

Fasting or caloric deprivation is a negative stress for the body. Therefore, the body will adapt to reduce this stress in the future. In other words, it will now store more fat—the only thing it can store in excess—than before. Both fat percentage and the number of fat-storing enzymes will increase when the normal diet is resumed.

Additionally, the body must get calories from some source to function normally. So the body switches to burning muscle tissue for the energy not supplied through the diet. Low-calorie dieters usually experience one pound of muscle loss with every pound of fat loss. Since 90% of the body's metabolism is in the muscle tissue, this muscle loss leads to a decrease in the amount of calories needed. Then, when a normal diet is resumed, dieters usually eat more calories than are required, and the amount of stored fat increases.

LOSING WEIGHT (FOR WRESTLING AND OTHER WEIGHT CLASS SPORTS)

Some sports, such as wrestling and some crew events, have strict weight classes. Athletes try to become as lean and light as possible so they can compete in a weight class where they will be most successful. Some wrestlers lose 3 to 20% of their pre-season body weight. Frequently, however, the reducing techniques involve food restriction, fluid deprivation and fluid loss through sweating, which is induced by intense exercise or thermal insulation (special suits that do not allow heat loss from the body and thereby cause excessive sweating). Unfortunately, most athletes choose dehydration as their source of weight loss.

Dehydration hinders athletic performance in many ways. Some of these include:

- Decreased muscular strength
- Decreased muscular endurance
- Decreased blood volume
- Decreased cardiac function at high heart rates
- Decreased oxygen uptake (especially with food restriction)
- Decreased glycogen storage
- Increased electrolyte loss.

Coaches should note that, although there is anywhere from one to five hours after weigh-in, that is not enough time to re-establish normal hydration levels. For these reasons, apply these rules for athletes at all times:

- Keep caloric intake up. Minimum intake should be between 1,200 and 2,400 **Kcalories**, or food calories, per day.

- Have body composition measured. Studies show that athletes' body fat should not drop below 5%. When their actual body fat percentage is determined, use the following equations to determine the amount of suitable fat—*not water*—loss.

$$\frac{\text{\% BODY FAT}}{100} \times \frac{\text{BODY WEIGHT}}{1} = \text{FAT WEIGHT}$$

$$\frac{\text{FAT WEIGHT}}{1} \times \frac{\text{\% BODY FAT - 5}}{\text{\% BODY FAT}} = \text{POUNDS TO LOSE} \quad (5)$$

ACTUAL WEIGHT-POUNDS TO LOSE = TARGET WEIGHT

- Discourage all dehydration techniques, especially before competition.
- Make sure that the athlete's target weight is reached three to four days before competition.

GAINING WEIGHT

A large body mass is a distinct advantage in many sports. There are many techniques for weight gain, but they all center on taking in more calories than are being used. Every weight-gain program should include a heavy weight-lifting program and adequate aerobic conditioning to ensure that all the weight gained is not fat.

Most weight-gain strategies involve eating a large volume of Kcalories. Meals should include large servings of meat, bread and starchy vegetables. Experts also recommend eating high-calorie snacks such as high-Kcalorie milkshakes and sandwiches between meals.

The body will gain weight and muscle mass easily until it reaches a maximum value. Athletes can expect a weight gain of one-and-a-half to two pounds per week during this period. When this plateau weight, referred to as the **set point**, is reached, however, the body will try to resist further weight gain. The set point can be increased only by consistently holding body weight a few pounds above the observed set point for an extended period of time. This allows the body to adapt its set point to a higher level and prepares the muscles and bones for the increased mass. During this set point adjustment, expected weight gain will drop to about one-half to two pounds per month. Athletes should include rigorous weight lifting in their training during this period to make sure the natural muscle-building hormones are fully active.

AMINO ACID AND WEIGHT-GAIN SUPPLEMENTS

While very expensive, supplements are valuable in weight-gain programs. They allow athletes to consume large amounts of Kcalories and protein without constantly stuffing themselves with food. Remember, all Kcalories and protein not immediately needed by the body will be stored as fat. So, to avoid this, supplements and meals should be taken in smaller amounts but with greater frequency.

Some athletes experience gastric discomfort when taking protein and amino acid supplements. This happens because the body has a harder time breaking down proteins and therefore must retain them longer in the stomach in the presence of harsh, acidic chemicals. If athletes suffer gastric irritation, they should either drink plenty of milk and water or discontinue use of the product.

High protein diets can also lead to considerable stress on the renal system because the by-products of protein metabolism must be eliminated by the kidneys. If athletes are ingesting large amounts of protein, they should also drink plenty of fluids. Any athlete with kidney problems should avoid these diets.

2.4 ANABOLIC STEROIDS AND OTHER SUPPLEMENTS

ANABOLIC STEROIDS

Anabolic steroids are chemicals that functionally resemble the male hormone testosterone. These steroids may either be extracted from human cadavers or other animals, or synthesized in the laboratory. In recent years, thousands of athletes have added steroids to their training program because of its anabolic properties. **Anabolism** refers to tissue synthesis, which equates to increased muscle mass. Most athletes want more muscle mass because it leads to increased speed, strength and power.

Steroids, however, present a very dangerous risk to athletes. First, steroids are usually purchased on the black market from makeshift Mexican laboratories. These steroids are impure about 90% of the time. There is no way to predict what chemicals are contaminating the steroids. These compounds could be toxic, cancer-causing or induce an allergic reaction that could lead to shock and possible death. Some black market steroids are really a water solution, called blanks, that have no anabolic properties whatsoever. Obviously, users are playing Russian roulette with their bodies.

Second, steroids can cause changes in liver function. This condition may lead to cholestatic hepatitis, which causes permanent liver damage. A decrease in high-density lipoproteins (HDL) is also common in steroid users. When HDL decreases, the ratio of HDL to LDL (low-density lipoprotein) increases, a condition directly related to heightened risk of cardiovascular disease. Athletes with high serum cholesterol levels or depressed HDL levels are especially endangered by this increased risk.

Third, since anabolic steroids stimulate tissue synthesis, any undetected or newly forming growths such as cancers will also grow at an increased rate, leading to decreased detection and treatment time for potentially terminal diseases.

Steroids also have androgenic properties which produce the secondary sex characteristics of the male. These include deepening of the voice, widening of the jaw, production of patterned body hair growth and enlargement of the gonads. These side effects are particularly noticeable and undesirable for females. Women who use steroids also suffer irregular or absent menstrual cycles, enlargement of the clitoris and atrophy of the breasts. Men also may experience acne, baldness, suppression of sperm production, prostate enlargement and genital atrophy. Both sexes frequently suffer decreased sex drive and water retention (bloating).

Steroids are particularly bad for adolescent athletes. They not only risk all the aforementioned side effects, but they also accelerate the closure of the epiphyseal growth plates, which can shorten bone length.

Although steroids produce desirable effects such as anabolism, the destructive potential of these drugs far outweighs the benefits. Steroids have many clinical uses in disease treatment, but their use in athletics should *never* be accepted or tolerated.

BLOOD DOPING

Blood doping involves increasing the red blood cell count by intravenous infusion. This infusion raises the hemoglobin level, allowing the blood to carry more oxygen, which seems to increase endurance. The safety of this procedure has been questioned by current research. Therefore, blood doping should never be considered in amateur athletics.

BICARBONATE LOADING

Bicarbonate is the major blood buffering system of the body. It helps maintain normal blood pH in the presence of increased carbon dioxide and lactic acid. Users add a bicarbonate solution to the blood through intravenous injection to increase the buffering potential. Increased blood buffering capacity allows anaerobic activity to continue longer, which would be beneficial in most athletic events. Again, this technique is not fully researched, and its use in amateur athletics should not be considered.

AMINO ACID AND MUSCLE GAINING SUPPLEMENTS

These supplements, which can have beneficial effects for some athletes and are discussed on page 68.

2.5 THE FEMALE ATHLETE

In recent years, the number of amateur female athletes has grown dramatically as women begin to realize their athletic potential.

Although there is currently a large strength discrepancy between males and females, studies show that females have very close to the same strength potential per body-weight pound as males. This current strength separation among the sexes is good reason to separate men and women in contact sports. Still, many youth programs allow females to compete in male-dominated leagues. This is a positive step for women's athletics. Today, females are starting to get involved in sports earlier than ever, and are improving their agility and coordination alongside extremely competitive male athletes. Coaches should not treat these female athletes differently, and should encourage them to train hard and be confident during competition.

The rate of injury seems to be identical among the sexes once equal conditioning is achieved. However, injuries do occur in different areas in women's athletics, compared to men, because the techniques and sports are often dissimilar.

From a Sports Medicine standpoint, female athletes should be encouraged to exercise and compete because it retards the natural hormonal tendencies of osteoporosis and obesity. Some female athletes may experience menstrual abnormalities such as increased menstrual irregularity, amenorrhea (absent menstrual cycles) and menarcheal delay (delay of onset of menstruation). These problems can be caused by weight loss, fat loss, dietary alteration, physical stress, emotional stress and hormone alterations.

During intense training, blood levels of luteinizing hormone and progesterone are decreased. The degree of hormone depression is closely related to the intensity of training and is therefore a response to the athletes' physical and mental stresses. This condition can lead to *temporary* sterility. Athletes should be examined by a physician if the athlete:

•Wishes to become pregnant
•Does not develop sexually before age 13
•Has not started menstruation before age 16.

Some female athletes prefer delayed menarche because it prolongs their pre-pubertal physique, delaying the fat-depositing or hip-widening influences of estrogen that sometimes hamper performance. Any athlete who wishes to become pregnant or has not developed sexually within a normal period of time, however, should be examined by a physician to rule out factors other than the stress of exercise. These factors might include faulty steroid biosynthesis, gonadal failure, CNS tumors, pituitary deficiencies or malnutrition.

Female athletes should be encouraged to participate during menstruation and premenstrual syndrome (PMS). Any pregnant athlete should consult a physician prior to training.

Female hormones and menstrual flow often make calcium and iron supplementation necessary. Under normal levels of estrogen, females need 1000 mg of calcium per day to decrease the potential for bone loss and subsequent osteoporosis. Similarly, women lose iron during menstrual flow, and female athletes sometimes require iron supplements between puberty and menopause to avoid anemia and related conditions. Female athletes also need increased levels of thiamin (B_1), riboflavin (B_2), niacin (B_3) and pantothenic acid, which are normally sufficiently supplied through a well-balanced diet. Always consult a physician to determine if any supplements are necessary.

2.6 THE DIABETIC ATHLETE

Diabetes is a disorder characterized by high blood sugar levels and excessive urination. The most common form of diabetes, **diabetes mellitus**, is characterized by a deficiency or inactive form of insulin. Symptoms include insatiable thirst, hunger, sugar in the urine, weakness from excessive leanness and coma. This condition must be treated by a special diet and/or insulin injections, both of which are under the control of a physician. Coaches should be aware of any athlete with this condition.

Diabetics may suffer from two blood sugar conditions, hypoglycemia and hyperglycemia. **Hypoglycemia**, or insulin shock, is caused by a deficiency of sugar in the blood. **Hyperglycemia** is caused by too much sugar in the blood. For more information on how these conditions affect athletes, see section 5.2.

3 Keys to Injury Prevention

Prevention of athletic injuries begins with pre-season training that shapes and strengthens players' bodies. It also includes warm-up exercises before every practice and game.

To paraphrase an old saying, "An ounce of prevention is worth four pounds of rehabilitation." Think of it this way: A star player begins practice without stretching and conditioning, then pulls a hamstring muscle in practice. The injury might have been prevented if the muscles were loose or in aerobic condition. If the coach had taken just 15 minutes out of the practice for prevention, an injury may have been prevented. Instead, he lost his most valuable player for three weeks. Although prevention will not stop all injuries, it can definitely reduce the chance of injury.

A good prevention program includes stretching and warm-up exercises.

3.1 STRETCHING

Stretching is a necessary part of daily body maintenance. It is beneficial for non-athletes and athletes alike. Stretching serves many purposes, including:

- Lengthening muscles after sleep or long relaxation
- Increasing blood flow into the muscles for nourishment and repair
- Preparing muscles for active movement, whether work or play
- Maintaining or increasing flexibility
- Increasing speed, agility and balance
- Warming down muscles after a workout to prevent tightening.

Coaches who incorporate good stretching programs into their workouts notice substantial improvement in athletic performance. Stretching also reduces the risk of injury.

Stretching must be done regularly and properly, however, to achieve an increase in flexibility. Consider the following suggestions for safe, effective stretching.

CORRECT STRETCHING

•Relax your whole body when stretching.

•Breathe comfortably and naturally while continually taking slow, deep breaths.

•Always hold a stretch in a comfortable position. Once you feel your body relax, increase the stretch without straining.

•Mentally feel the stretch; think about the muscles you are stretching. If the tension in the muscles becomes too great, back off the stretch into a consistent, comfortable tension.

•You should stretch at least once a day, and three or four times daily, if possible.

•Stretching should be approached with a positive attitude; it is healthy for your body and makes you feel good!

•Make stretching fun and painless. Do it properly, and the reward of flexibility will come with time.

INCORRECT STRETCHING

•Never bounce when stretching. Bouncing causes a reflex action in your muscles and tightens the very muscles you are trying to loosen.

•Never overstretch. Overstretching can damage muscle tissues, thus doing more harm than good. If stretching is painful, it may indicate that you are overstretching or stretching incorrectly.

- Never compare yourself with others. Everyone's body is different, and someone else's flexibility has nothing to do with your flexibility.

10-MINUTE FULL BODY STRETCH

Illustrations of the movements are shown at the end of this section.

Underlined items refer to specific muscles and/or muscle groups.

AREA STRETCHED	STRETCH PROCEDURE
1. BACK, HIPS, UPPER BODY	While keeping the feet and ankles in the forward position, rotate the entire rest of the body to the left and then to the right as far as is comfortable. Start very slow and increase slowly when loose. Repeat 10 times.
2. CERVICAL SPINE (NECK)	Roll head along shoulder area in slow, very exaggerated revolutions.
3. TRICEPS, LATERAL ABDOMINALS	Place right arm in back of neck as shown. With the left hand, pull the right elbow downward. Then switch arms and repeat.
4. SHOULDER, UPPER BACK, & CHEST	Clasp hands behind back and pull arms up to a comfortable stretch. Someone may pull the arms up, or a chair may be used. Tilt head back for added stretch.

5. LUMBAR AREA, GROIN, HAMSTRING	Sit with legs spread, and knees and palms on the ground. Bend entire body forward, trying to eventually touch the chest to the ground.
6. GROIN, SPINAL MUSCLES	Pull in heels as far as possible toward groin area. Put hands on feet and elbows on knees. Push down on knees with elbows, tuck head to chest, and lean upper body forward.
7. LOWER BACK	Lie on the floor with hands underneath chest. Push up with hands, leaving hips on the ground. Tilt head toward ceiling, and arch back.
8. TRAPEZIUS, HAMSTRINGS	Bend one leg so the foot touches the opposite knee, while the other leg is straight in front of body. For 15 seconds, stretch hamstrings by extending arms and chin toward the extended foot and leaning forward. For the next 15 seconds, stretch trapezius and spinal area by tucking chin to chest, rolling shoulders forward, and leaning toward extended foot.

9. QUADRICEPS	Tuck one leg back toward the posterior. Bend the other leg in an anterior position with the foot touching the opposite knee (see diagram). Slowly lower the body back until reaching a comfortable stretch.
10. LATERAL QUADRICEPS, GLUTEALS, SPINAL MUSCLES	Cross one leg over the other. Turn body the opposite way of the crossed leg (see diagram). Look straight behind and place free arm directly behind body. With the elbow on the bent knee, apply pressure in the opposite direction. Switch directions.
11. SHINS, KNEE, QUADRICEPS	Sit on the floor as shown in diagram #11. Be sure toes are pointed toward posterior. Slowly lower upper body backward, using arms as a brace to hold the position at desired stretch.
12. NECK, SPINE	Lie on floor with feet slightly spread and knees slightly bent. Place hands behind head and raise until a stretch is felt down spine.

13. <u>ACHILLES TENDON, SOLEUS</u>	Lean against a wall with front leg bent. Make sure both feet are pointed directly forward. For 15 seconds, push hips toward the wall without lifting heels and without bending the back knee. For the next 15 seconds, bend back knee slightly, and stretch forward again without lifting heels.
14. ANKLES	While sitting on the floor, hold an ankle in the air and, with the other hand, rotate the ankle through its entire range of motion 10 times or until ankle is loose.

figure 3-1. A ten minute stretching program. Directions can be found on the previous pages.

10-MINUTE STRETCHING PROGRAM

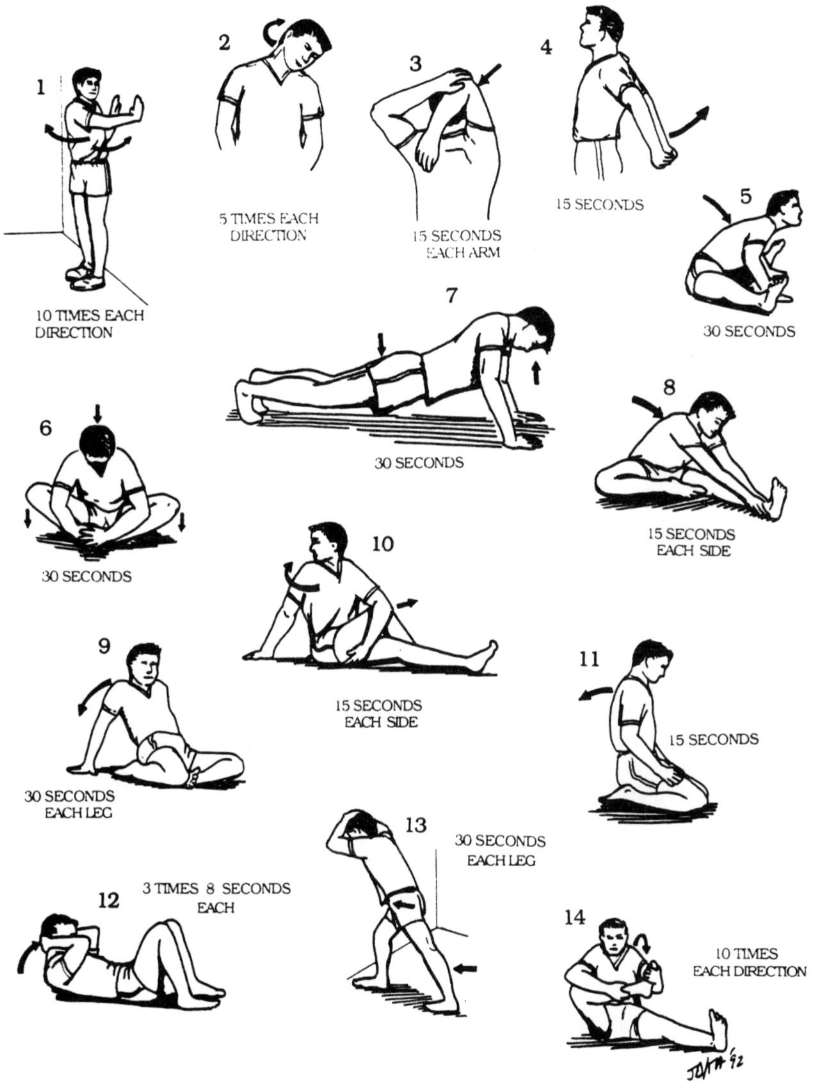

3.2 WARM-UP EXERCISES

Calisthenics warm up the joints and muscles. These exercises should vary somewhat depending upon the sport. Here's a sample routine:

1. Light jogging
2. Stretching
3. Jumping jacks
4. High knee raises—jogging in place
5. Arm rotations
6. Backward running
7. Slow takeoffs from stance
8. Acceleration runs.

3.3 ACCLIMATION OF ATHLETES

There are four environmental factors that significantly influence athletic performance: heat, cold, humidity and altitude. The production and loss of heat, the transport of oxygen and nutrients, and water retention and loss are directly related to the stresses of the environment. It is important to learn how the body reacts to the different environmental conditions to prevent illness. The best treatment for environmentally related illness is always prevention.

THE EFFECTS OF HEAT

The body's internal **core temperature** has a very narrow range of fluctuation within which the body can function properly. A loss or gain of a mere four degrees Fahrenheit can seriously hamper the regulation of certain body systems. Yet countless chemical reactions that control all vital bodily functions produce heat, and certain temperatures are needed for these chemical reactions to occur. If the core temperature is too hot, chemical reactions can accelerate out of control. If the temperature is too cold, reactions can halt altogether. During periods of strenuous activity, the body produces six to ten times more heat than the body does at rest. This heat buildup, which is often accompanied by high environmental temperatures, places a major stress on the body to alleviate the excess heat. Heat from the environment hinders the heat release systems of the body and can often increase the body's core temperature.

The body has four methods of dissipating heat from the body: radiation, convection, conduction, and sweating or evaporation. **Radiation** is the natural release of infrared rays from the skin's pores. If the outside temperature is much greater than the body's core temperature or if the body is surrounded by surfaces such as metal, snow, etc. that reflect infrared rays, the body's heat radiation is greatly decreased. **Convection** is cooling by currents of air that come in contact with the skin. Heat accumulated at the skin's surface is carried away. Wind boosts this heat dissipation system. **Conduction** is the direct transfer of heat from a warmer body to a cooler body. If, for instance, you touch an ice cube, the heat is transferred from your hand into the ice. When the previous three cooling methods are insufficient or unavailable, the body has no choice but to activate the **sweating/evaporation process**. Sweat from the sweat glands can cool an athlete under most circumstances. Sweat that touches the skin and then evaporates dissipates a tremendous amount of heat. There are limits to this system, however. If this process is disrupted, an athlete can suffer serious and even fatal heat illness.

Always know and follow these rules to avoid problems with *heat*:

- Use white, light or bright-colored clothing for practice and game uniforms.
- Constantly drink cool water.
- Acclimate athletes to hot weather slowly by gradually increasing workout activities.
- Change practice times to mornings or evenings, when temperatures are lower.
- Monitor weight loss. If athletes lose 3 to 5% of their body weight, they should be removed from competition until the weight is regained.
- Keep skin moist and allow sufficient recuperation time between drills.

- Monitor susceptible athletes. Obese, heavily muscled or unacclimated athletes are especially susceptible.

THE EFFECTS OF COLD

Exercise in cold weather requires considerable preventive measures to ensure safe play. Cold temperatures slow all body functions, including metabolism. Muscles also contract to conserve heat, which causes considerable tightness. An inner core temperature of less than 96 degrees Fahrenheit indicates the body is losing its ability to retain enough heat and is falling into **hypothermia**, or too little heat. Hypothermia, a life-threatening condition, and **frostbite**, which is frozen, dying tissue in the extremities, can be prevented by adhering to certain rules when playing in cold climates.

Always know and follow these rules to avoid problems with *cold*:

- Increase your calisthenic program to at least 30 minutes.

- Require warm clothing and especially protection for areas of major heat loss (head, hands, feet, etc.).

- Encourage athletes to drink water constantly, even if they do not feel thirsty.

- Have players replace wet clothing as soon as possible. Athletes can bring spare clothes if conditions are bad.

- Have athletes jog and stretch constantly on the sidelines.

- If an athlete:
  - Shivers excessively
  - Has bluish-red, hard skin on face, feet, or toes
  - Is sluggish
  - Has body temperature of 96 degrees or below

REMOVE FROM COMPETITION AND WARM IMMEDIATELY.

THE EFFECTS OF HUMIDITY

High humidity is one of the major causes of heat illness because it greatly slows heat dissipation. At humidity levels of 75% or more, sweating has little or no cooling effect. Sweat on the skin cannot evaporate because of the high percent of water vapor in the air, so sweating only leads to dehydration.

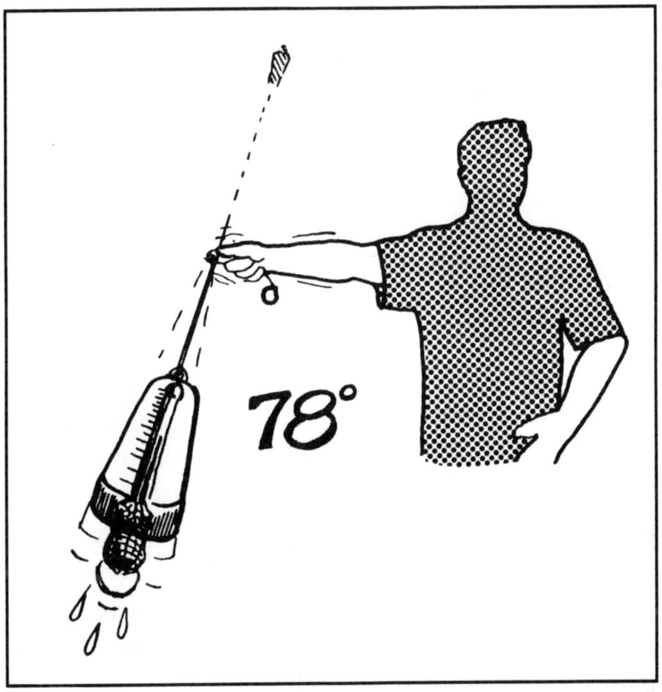

figure 3-2. The wet bulb test measures the combined effects of temperature and humidity. A reading of 78° or higher indicates unsafe playing conditions.

Always know and follow these rules to avoid problems with *humidity*:

- Use the wet bulb test to measure the com bined effects of temperature and humidity. A reading of 78 degrees or above indicates dangerous playing conditions, and the athletic event should be canceled.
- Acclimate athletes slowly to a humid climate.
- Provide water before, during and after practice.
- Allow athletes frequent breaks either in the shade or a cooled area.

THE EFFECTS OF ALTITUDE

In high altitude locations, the air is much thinner. The percentage of oxygen in the air remains the same, but the atmospheric pressure is much lower than at sea level. This decrease in pressure does not force the oxygen molecules across the lung membranes as efficiently, making oxygen uptake more difficult. To make up for this, the body responds by increasing the respiratory rate as well as the number of red blood cells (which means more hemoglobin). This acclimation takes time, and coaches should recognize this period characterized by decreased aerobic capacity. The normal adjustment time for athletes is 4 to 14 days, depending on the altitude and the temperature.

3.4 AGILITY AND COORDINATION

Agility is the ability to move body parts quickly and accurately. This ability takes considerable coordination, or synchronization, of the nervous and muscular systems. Since both of these qualities must be developed through training, they are both *learned* skills. Athletes should start exercising the mind and body together at an early age since these attributes are desirable in *every* athletic event.

You can teach young athletes hand-eye coordination through ball tossing and catching, craft construction and other dexterous activities. In fact, this might be one of the few positive aspects of playing video games.

Athletes also need to develop foot quickness. They should be taught to be "light on their feet" and be able to change directions quickly during a full sprint. Many coaches use drills such as running through tires, shuttle runs and other drills in which the feet are moving as rapidly as possible and a change in direction is necessary.

During their adolescent years, athletes who have already received agility training have a distinct advantage over untrained teammates because they have better control over their rapidly growing bodies and, consequently, have less chance of injury.

3.5 WEIGHT TRAINING

Weight lifting often helps prevent athletic injuries, although it should never be done without proper instruction and stretching. Athletes who lift weight must be especially careful at all times because of the strong forces applied to the muscles and tendons. Lifts that involve only one muscle group, which receives all the weight and torque, require particular caution.

Weight training increases the strength and size of the muscle fibers. This is because the muscle fibers are stressed when the force of the weight is greater than the force of resistance generated by the muscles. In anticipation of confronting this force again, the body repairs the muscle fibers so they are larger and stronger than before. This process of muscle enlargement is called **hypertrophy**. If the muscles are not continually subjected to the large force of weights, the body will break down the muscles to the size they were before the weight training program. This process of muscle reduction is called **atrophy**, and can only be avoided by continually stressing the muscle tissue.

There are various types of weight training equipment available, each with its advantages and disadvantages:

- **Free weights** provide a constant force throughout the ROM, or range of motion.

This approach allows a large amount of force to be applied on the fibers and produces the greatest amount of hypertrophy. Since the weights are not attached to pulleys or other restrictive machines, free weights allow other muscle groups to balance and stabilize the body parts that are being exercised. This type of lifting closely resembles the forces encountered during athletic competition because balance and stabilization are involved.

- **Universal weight** machines use the force of gravity as an additional resistive force by only allowing the weight to be moved vertically.

To accomplish this, the weights are stacked and lifted along a guide bar by a pulley system (figure 3-3). These machines enable athletes to exercise many muscle groups without a lot of equipment. Since the weight is confined to a pulley system, however, the balance and stabilization forces are greatly reduced and the ROM is limited.

• **Variable resistance** training, the sort provided by Nautilus™ equipment, maintains equal force on the muscles during the entire ROM.

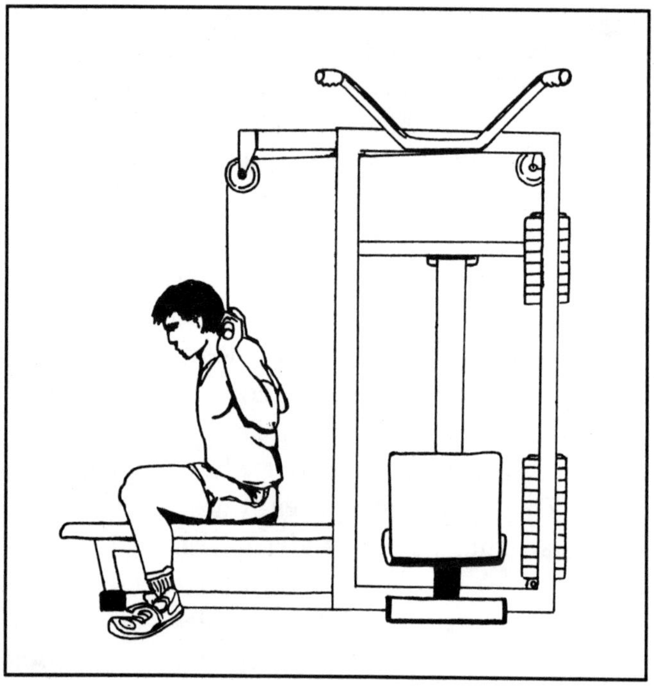

figure 3-3. Weight training using Universal type equipment.

This equal force is not possible with the other techniques because muscles cannot generate the same amount of force at all joint angles. Variable resistance machines use an irregularly shaped pulley to constantly change the force of the machine to match the differing strength angles of the muscles. These machines become costly because a different machine is needed for each exercise.

Weight lifting should be done every other day since muscles require at least 48 hours to rebuild after strength training sessions. Some athletes stagger their workouts to exercise certain body parts every third or fourth day. Using this technique, an athlete can lift every day, letting some muscles heal while exercising others. This approach also greatly reduces the time spent in the gym and maximizes strength gain, but the athlete or coach needs to combine muscle groups that are responsible for related movements. As an example, group the chest and triceps, which are responsible for pushing motion, on one day, and group the biceps and latissimus dorsi, which are the pulling muscles, the next day.

Start each lift with a warm-up set, such as bench pressing 100 pounds 10 times before lifting 160 pounds. This is very important because it increases blood flow and warms up the muscles and tendons. Athletes should start at a low, comfortable weight and increase a little at each workout. The largest muscle group should be exercised first. So, the hip and thigh muscle group would usually precede a smaller group, such as the biceps and triceps in the arms. Alternating muscle groups will allow other groups to recover between the various lifting sets.

Athletes who wish to gain muscle mass, strength and power should lift heavy weights with fewer repetitions. Athletes who want to tone, define or increase muscle endurance should lift lighter weights with many repetitions.

Muscles are only strengthened at the angles they are exercised, so always lift through the full range of motion. Weight lifting is not a relaxing workout like stretching, however, lifters should still exercise good judgment and not push themselves beyond their personal limit. If a lifter becomes disoriented or experiences pain in any joints, the lifting program should be re-evaluated. Weight lifters should be supervised at all times by a coach or spotter and should never be left unattended even for five minutes.

The issue of weight training for children is controversial (also see p. 38). The most generally accepted method of improving children's muscular strength and endurance is using their natural body weight with calisthenic exercises. Younger children can take part in a weight program to learn coordination, but not to bulk up. To learn coordination, children can use just the weight of the bar to lift through the entire range of motion. Remember, the emphasis of sports for children should be learning, developing sports skills, and most of all, having fun!

A weight-lifting program can serve as a valuable tool for conditioning athletes and strengthening their bodies. Always keep in mind: "An hour of prevention is worth four days of rehabilitation."

Athletes should always follow these weight-lifting rules:

- Lifters should always stretch before and after lifting.

- Lifters should wear proper clothing and protective equipment, including belts and gloves.

- Lifters should always have a spotter nearby.

- Do not participate in or allow horseplay in the weight room because of the high potential for accidents.

- Be sure you are lifting the correct way and are in the proper position. If you have any questions, ask the coach.

****SEE APPENDIX FOR ILLUSTRATIONS OF COMMON WEIGHT TRAINING EXERCISES*****

3.6 PREVENTIVE TAPING

Taping a joint, such as the ankle or the wrist, as a preventive precaution, is usually not necessary. Instead, the surrounding muscles, tendons and ligaments that would be supported by the tape should be strengthened with conditioning exercises. If an injury does occur, an athlete should spend sufficient time rehabilitating the weakened joint before applying any tape. Once they regain full strength, the tape should not be used to support the joint. To protect previously injured joints such as elbows and knees, braces may be recommended to prevent further damage to the medial and lateral ligaments.

Taping is generally used for supporting a chronic weakness or a joint that has not had enough rehabilitation to strengthen to its full capacity. Section 7.5 offers further information on taping.

4 Coaching at the Amateur Level

A coach is a leader and an organizer as well as a teacher, and therefore must command the respect of athletes. At the same time, players have certain rights, too. Coaches should respect their players, and nothing should dampen this mutual admiration. Nonetheless, amateur sports is a learning situation in which emotions can become unstable. Players are often sensitive about criticism, so it is absolutely critical for the coach to help preserve the athletes' pride and maintain their morale because psychological stress and anxiety can discourage anyone. *Remember, as a coach, you are the athlete's friend as well as a teacher.*

This chapter includes tips for coaches as well as athletes and parents.

4.1 THE COACH

Coaches have a tremendous responsibility to their athletes, their programs and themselves. To fulfill these responsibilities and the promise they hold, they must be properly educated and prepared.

THE COACH'S EDUCATION

Amateur coaches should be educated in the following disciplines:

1. CPR
2. Basic first aid
3. Basic Sports Medicine (if the program is available)
4. Specifics of the sport they are coaching.

Coaches are expected to perform to the best of their abilities. If they are educated in these four areas, coaches have little legal risk. Such knowledge far outweighs the value of a certification card.

Another legal protection is the **Good Samaritan Laws**, which were developed for volunteers who act on their own goodwill. These laws, which differ from community to community and state to state, grant you immunity from liability if you act in good faith to provide emergency care to the level of your training and to the best of your ability. Become familiar with your local and state laws in the unfortunate case you may need to know them.

THE COACH AS TEACHER

The nature of athletic competition requires players to be educated in many areas. Since coaches are responsible for this education, they must have the athletes' respect and trust as well as an understanding of the game and proper training techniques. In their role as teachers, coaches should share the important information in this manual to increase their athletes' understanding of their own bodies. For example, it is not important for an athlete to understand the general injury procedure, but it *is* important for them to know not to move a player with a probable neck injury. Furthermore, it is important for athletes to understand what is appropriate to eat before competition, but they do not need to memorize the four food groups.

** Remember, it is the coaches' responsibility to produce a team that is safe as well as competitive, and to insure the athletes' proper mental and physical growth. **

THE COACHES' CODE OF ETHICS

I. I will treat each player, opposing coach, official, parent and administrator with respect and dignity.

II. I will do my best to learn the fundamental skills, teaching and evaluation techniques, and strategies of my sport.

III. I will become thoroughly familiar with the rules of my sport.

IV. I will become familiar with the objectives of the youth sports program with which I am affiliated. I will strive to achieve these objectives and communicate them to my players and their parents.

V. I will uphold the authority of officials who are assigned to the contests in which I coach, and I will assist them in every way to conduct fair and impartial competitive contests and *never* question their judgment.

VI. I will learn the strengths and weakness of my players so that I might place them into situations in which they have a maximum opportunity to achieve success.

VII. I will conduct my practices and games so that all players have an opportunity to improve their skill level through active participation.

VIII. I will communicate to my players and their parents the rights and responsibilities of individuals on our team.

IX. I will cooperate with the administrator of our organization in the enforcement of rules and regulations, and I will report any irregularities that violate sound competitive practices.

X. I will protect the health and safety of my players by insisting that all of the activities under my control are conducted for their psychological and physiological welfare, rather than for the vicarious interests of adults.

Reprinted from an article which appeared in Spotlight on Youth Sports, *Vol. 2, 1979 entitled "Young Athletes Have a Bill of Rights, Do We Need a Code Of Ethics for Coaches?" by Vern Seefeldt.*

THE COACH'S DUTIES

There are many responsibilities inherent in the coaching position. A coach's first task is to become educated in the four areas listed in the introduction to this section. Second, you must plan your coaching strategy. This includes planning all practices from start to finish, scheduling games (if appropriate) and bringing the proper equipment to each event.

Although this is not a complete list of coaching responsibilities, these guidelines should be followed by all coaches at all times:

1. Be in complete control of the team at all times: supervise stretching, warm-ups, pre-game meals, curfews, etc.

2. Carry the **Coach's Kit** (included in this chapter) to every practice or game. Be sure the Consent for Treatment Forms, Medical Questionnaire, clipboard and all first aid supplies are present.

3. *Always* carry 25 cents in your pocket to call for an ambulance or professional medical assistance in case of emergency. (You may also dial 911 where the service is available.)

4. Know where the closest phone is located.

5. Inspect the field. Note access for emergency vehicles, locked gates, holes in the field, bumps or any other obstacles that may cause harm to the athletes.

6. Make sure a water source is near, or bring water and cups to every event.

7. Line the fields with flour or a similar material. Lime causes terrible irritation to the eyes if an athlete slides into it.

8. Shorten practices when temperatures and humidity are high (see section 3.3 on Acclimation). You do not need to be accountable for an athlete's death because of heat stroke or dehydration.

9. Allow proper warm-up and cool-down times. Allow at least 20 minutes for stretching and warm-ups and at least 10 minutes for cool-down stretching and jogging.

10. Use common sense, and do not push the athletes beyond reasonable limits.

Somatotyping

One of a coach's many responsibilities is matching athletes with the best sport or position for that particular person. Coaches often use **somatotyping** (see figure 4.1) to determine athletes overall body shape and structure, and to gain a rough idea of their body composition.

All humans fit into one of three categories: ectomorphs, endomorphs and mesomorphs. **Ectomorphs** are characterized by their tall, thin frames. Their bodies usually carry little body fat and musculature. Many basketball players and long distance runners are ectomorphs. **Endomorphs** usually have short, thick frames. They carry considerable fat and muscle and are often obese. Athletes with this body type often become football linemen or participate in field sports such as shotput and discus. Finally, **mesomorphs** have the typical athletic, medium frame that can carry considerable muscle. Their bodies are usually rather lean and toned. Most athletes fit into this category, and mesomorphs are therefore found in every sport.

It is important to realize that somatotyping does not use height and aerobic conditioning as key characteristics. For example, a very thin wrestler

figure 4-1. The three somatotype classifications.

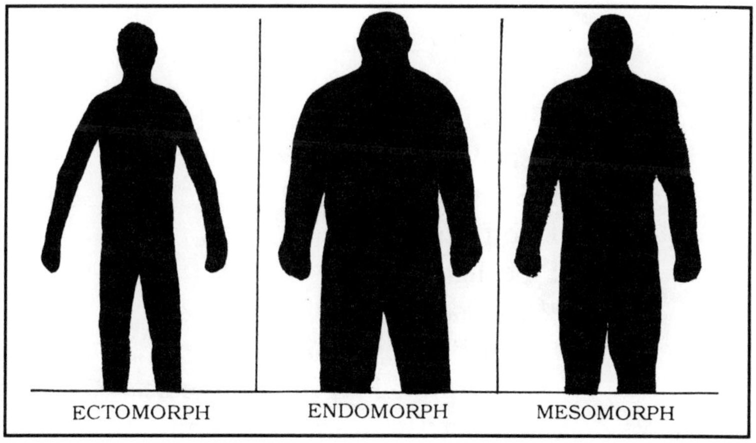

standing 5'4" and weighing 90 pounds would most likely fit into the ectomorph category even though he is not tall. Similarly, an endomorphic lineman may be in better cardiovascular shape than any other member of the team.

On the other hand, strength potential strongly correlates to body type. Generally, larger body types exhibit more strength potential, although there are exceptions.

THE COACH'S KIT

A coach should have the following materials present at *all* athletic events:

1 cold (chemical) pack or plastic bags for ice
1 pair taping scissors
2 rolls athletic tape
1 roll pre-wrap
2 4" elastic wrap bandages
4 tongue depressors (for finger splints)
1 folded strip of cardboard (splint)
1 arm sling
6 pairs surgical gloves
3 butterfly bandages
4 different sized bandages
4 sterile pads
2 alcohol swabs
4 4" x 4" gauze pads
1 coach's clipboard
1 whistle
1 quarter (25 cents)
1 eyewash
1 small bottle of tincture of benzoin
1 small bottle of hydrogen peroxide
1 Swiss Army knife
1 soft mouthpiece
1 penlight
•*Handbook of Sports Medicine*
•A complete player roster
•*All* Return to Play Forms, Medical Release forms, Medical Questionnaire and other medical records, 5" x 7" cards
•CPR, basic first aid and other relevant certification cards

Be sure to restock the kit when items are used!

This kit is the coach's most valuable possession. The kit not only provides first aid equipment, but also provides a place for the coach to organize and carry the player rosters and game plan so they are not forgotten on game day.

These forms (which are in the next section), along with up-to-date medical records, are a coach's ultimate protection from legal responsibility. Coaches should *require* all participating athletes to fill out the Medical Release/Medical Questionnaire *before* the first day of practice. Coaches should also *require* all athletes who are unable to play for an extended period of time to get the Return to Play Form signed by a physician *before* returning to practice. If this process is not followed, the coach holds legal responsibility.

As a general rule, coaches should take all possible steps to clear themselves from liability and to prepare themselves for unexpected events. This includes exercising good judgment when dealing with the athletes. Don't let injured athletes play, even if they demand it or a championship depends on it. Coaches must always remember that youth athletics is a recreational activity, and its main purpose is *fun*, not winning.

LEGAL AND MEDICAL FORMS

The following pages contain legal and medical release forms that you may reproduce and use.

MEDICAL RELEASE FOR MINOR CHILD

I, ______________________________, Parent or Legal Guardian of ________________________ a minor child, hereby authorize any Medical or Surgical treatment which may be necessary in an emergency, and in my absence, for the well being of the above mentioned minor. I agree to hold the physician or hospital treating the above mentioned minor, harmless.

____________________ has the following allergies:

________________________and has the following medical

conditions: ______________________________

____

Dated________________ Signed____________________

Parent or Legal Guardian

RETURN TO PLAY FORM

THIS SECTION TO BE FILLED OUT BY THE ATHLETE

1. PERSONAL INFORMATION

Name of Athlete______________________________ Age:_______

Position Played/Sport_____________________________________

School/Organization_______________________________________

Home Phone _______________Parents' Work Phone ____________

2. INJURY INFORMATION

Date of Injury_________________

Injured in (check one) Practice___Game___Other________________

Brief description on how injury occurred______________________

____

THIS SECTION TO BE COMPLETED BY PHYSICIAN

PLEASE CALL OR ALLOW THE ATHLETE TO RETURN THE RESULTS OF THIS FORM TO HIS/HER COACH. THANK YOU.

3. Description of injury____________________________________

____

4. RECOMMENDATIONS FOR TREATMENT AT SCHOOL

(check one or more)

_____Cold Packs _____Cold Whirlpool

_____Moist Heat/Whirlpool _____Other

5. FURTHER RECOMMENDATIONS (please check one or more)

____Referred to____

____No Practice or Play Until____________________________(date)

____No Restrictions (Discharged as of)___________________(date)

____Light Running Only

____Regular Practice (No Contact)

____Other__________________________________

Physician______________________Date________Phone_______________

MEDICAL QUESTIONNAIRE

Name_______________________________Phone_________________
Address__________________________________Birthdate___________
FamilyPhysican_______________________Phone_________________

WHO TO CONTACT IN CASE OF EMERGENCY:
Name__________________________________Phone_____________
Relationship to you____

HAVE YOU HAD OR DO YOU NOW HAVE ANY OF THE FOLLOWING:

*****If YES, please specify below*****

Hernia	Yes_____	No_____
Diabetes	Yes_____	No_____
Heart murmur	Yes_____	No_____
Allergies	Yes_____	No_____
Injuries to joints:		
Shoulder	Yes_____	No_____
Knee	Yes_____	No_____
Ankle	Yes_____	No_____
Fingers	Yes_____	No_____
Other	Yes_____	No_____
Frequent earaches	Yes_____	No_____
Diarrhea	Yes_____	No_____
Poor vision	Yes_____	No_____
Poor hearing	Yes_____	No_____

HAVE YOU HAD A RECENT
TETANUS BOOSTER? Yes_____ No_____ When?__________

ARE YOU CURRENTLY TAKING
ANY MEDICATION? Yes_____ No_____

If YES, what and why?____

DID YOUR DOCTOR PLACE ANY RESTRICTION ON YOUR
ATHLETIC ACTIVITY? Explain.
____
____
____

Signed:____
Parent's signature:_______________________________

4.2 THE ATHLETE

Athletes have many demands placed upon them by coaches, supporters and especially themselves. Young athletes feel the additional need to please their parents. For them to get the most out of their sports participation, everyone involved should observe the Young Athletes' Bill of Rights.

YOUNG ATHLETES' BILL OF RIGHTS

I. We have the right to participate in sports.

II. We each have the right to participate at a level commensurate with our own amount of maturity and ability.

III. We have the right to qualified adult leadership.

IV. We have the right to play as children, not adults.

V. We have the right to share in the leadership and decision-making about our sports participation.

VI. We have the right to participate in safe and healthy environments.

VII. We have the right to proper preparation for sports participation.

VIII. We have the right to equal opportunity to strive for success.

IX. We have the right to be treated with dignity.

X. We have the right to have fun in sports.

XI. We do not publicly question officials' judgments and *never* question their honesty.

From Fair Play Codes for Children in Sport, *Canadian Council on Children and Youth.*

4.3 THE PARENTS

Parents have a special responsibility in their children's athletic pursuits. To fulfill this responsibility, they must abide by their own set of rules.

THE PARENT'S CODE

I. Do not force an unwilling child to participate in sports.

II. Remember that children are involved in organized sports for their own enjoyment, not yours.

III. Encourage your child to always play by the rules.

IV. Teach your child that honest effort is as important as victory so that the result of each competition is accepted without undue disappointment.

V. Turn defeat to victory by helping your child work toward improving skill and good sportsmanship. Never ridicule or yell at your child for making a mistake or losing a competition.

VI. Remember that children learn best by example. Applaud good plays by your team *and* by members of the opposing team.

VII. Do not publicly question officials' judgments or their honesty.

VIII. Support all efforts to remove verbal and physical abuse from children's sporting activities.

IX. Recognize the value and importance of volunteer coaches. They give their time and resources to provide recreation activities for your child.

From Fair Play Codes for Children in Sport, *Canadian Council on Children and Youth.*

UNIT 2

SPORTS MEDICINE MEDICAL REFERENCE

Now that you have a good foundation in how and why the human body works, you are better equipped to handle emergency or injury situations. Some of those incidents are specific, such as a torn eyelid, while others affect the entire body.

Begin by studying Chapter 5, which details conditions that can affect the entire body. After you are familiar with these situations, you can use the Quick Reference Injury Guide inside the front cover when problems arise.

5 General First Aid

This chapter covers general conditions that affect the whole body. They appear in alphabetical order for the purpose of study. Whether you are a coach, an athlete or both, you will want to read and thoroughly understand this chapter *before* an emergency arises.

Then, should you face a problem on or off the field, you will have an invaluable, immediate grasp of the situation. Since we all know *seconds count* in emergencies, this basic understanding could mean the difference between success in or the end of an athletic career, or even life and death.

5.1 BLEEDING

Serious bleeding is life-threatening and should be controlled immediately. There are four different techniques to control bleeding:

1. Direct pressure
2. Elevation
3. Pressure points
4. Tourniquets.

SIGNS/SYMPTOMS:

- •Obvious bleeding (external)
- •Possible blue/red discoloration of skin or swelling (internal bleeding).

TECHNIQUE FOR TREATMENT:

** *Always wear surgical gloves when dealing with open wounds to protect against diseases that can be transmitted by blood, such as AIDS and hepatitis.* **

Direct Pressure/Elevation

1. Use direct pressure by placing hand with a cloth directly over injury site and pressing

*Treatments continued on next page

firmly against the wound. If the cloth fills with blood, *DO NOT REMOVE* it. Add a clean cloth on top of the soaked one.

2. While applying direct pressure at the injury site, elevate the wound above the level of the heart.

** DO NOT elevate injured area if a fracture or a serious internal injury is suspected. **

3. Treat for shock.

4. Once bleeding is controlled, cover the area with a sterile bandage.

Pressure Points

Pressure points can only be used to treat an injured extremity. They are effective only when used correctly, which begins with locating the proper pressure points.

figure 5-1. Locations of pressure points for arms (A) and legs (B).

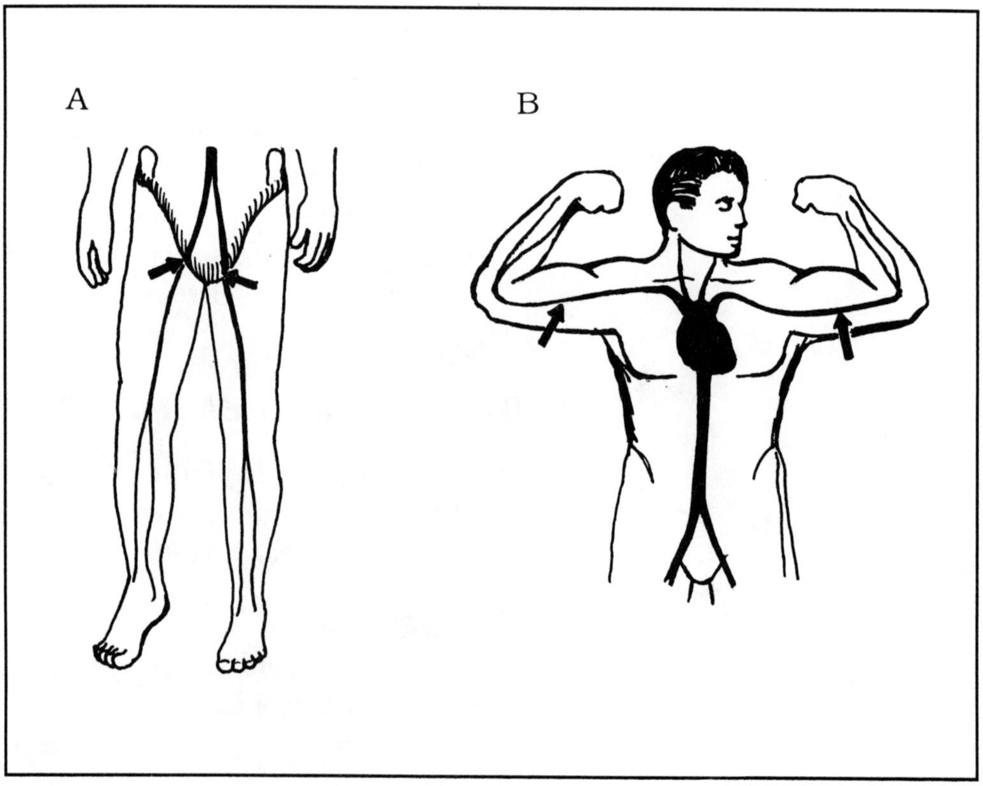

ARM

Squeeze fingers over the brachial artery, which is found on the medial side of the upper arm, halfway between the elbow and armpit. Squeeze with the length of your fingers toward your thumb and pull back on the artery while using the direct pressure technique at the injury site.

LEG

Use the heel of your hand to place firm pressure on the femoral artery, which is located on the *crease* between the leg and the torso. Provide firm pressure by using some body weight, and continue using direct pressure technique at the injury site.

Tourniquet

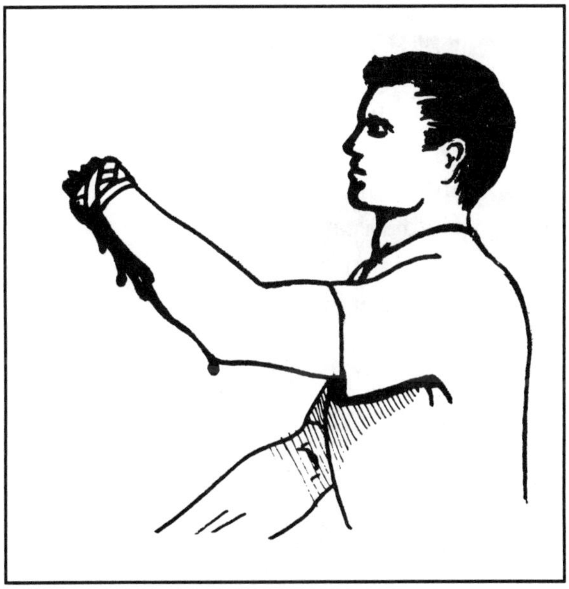

figure 5-2. Application of a tourniquet.

Tourniquets should only be used as a last resort after pressure and elevation have proven unsuccessful and an extremity can be sacrificed to save a victim's life (i.e., an amputation).

1. Place tourniquet as close to the wound as possible between the heart and the injured area.

2. Tighten tourniquet to stop *all* bleeding.

3. *CALL AN AMBULANCE.*

4. Pin a note with date, time and location of tourniquet on the victim.

5. Leave extremity with tourniquet exposed, but cover body to prevent shock.

5.2 BLOOD SUGAR ABNORMALITIES (DIABETES)

HYPOGLYCEMIA (TOO LITTLE SUGAR)

Hypoglycemia, or insulin shock, is caused by a deficiency of sugar in the blood. This condition might happen after an overdose of injected insulin, because the person has not eaten after an injection, or because of any harsh or unusual exercise or other psychological stresses. Children are especially susceptible to insulin shock.

SIGNS/SYMPTOMS:

•Continual hunger
•Dizziness
•Jittery feeling
•Cold sweat
•Tremor of the hands
•Dimness of vision
•Weakness
•Upset stomach
•Fainting.

TECHNIQUE FOR TREATMENT:

1. *RAISE BLOOD SUGAR QUICKLY.* Administer food, especially high sugar food such as sugar, candy, soft drinks, fruit juice, etc. *in small portions.*

2. If victim does not respond readily or is unconscious, call paramedics or quickly transport to emergency room. If possible, alert emergency room personnel that an unconscious diabetic will be arriving.

HYPERGLYCEMIA (TOO MUCH SUGAR)

Hyperglycemia refers to an excess of sugar in the blood. This may be caused by an inadequate or inactive insulin injection, yet also sometimes affects people who are unaware of their diabetic condition.

SIGNS/SYMPTOMS:

•Confusion
•Disorientation
•Drowsiness
•Deep, rapid breathing
•Breath with fruity odor
•Unconsciousness.

TECHNIQUE FOR TREATMENT:

Call paramedics or transport quickly to emergency room.

5.3 FAINTING

If brief faintness occurs without apparent injuries, have athlete lay down. Maintain normal body temperature. If athlete still feels faint or drifts into unconsciousness again, transport to emergency room. Constantly monitor ABCs (see section 6.1).

5.4 FRACTURES

A partial crack or complete break in a bone is called a fracture. Fractures can be open, or compound, with bone ends protruding through the skin, or closed, with the crack underneath skin.

SIGNS/SYMPTOMS:

•Difference in shape and length of corresponding body parts
•Obvious deformities, angulation or rotation of an extremity
•Open wound with visible bone protruding
•Localized pain and joint tenderness
•Swelling
•A pop or snap
•Reddish/blue skin discoloration
•Loss of movement and function of involved body part.

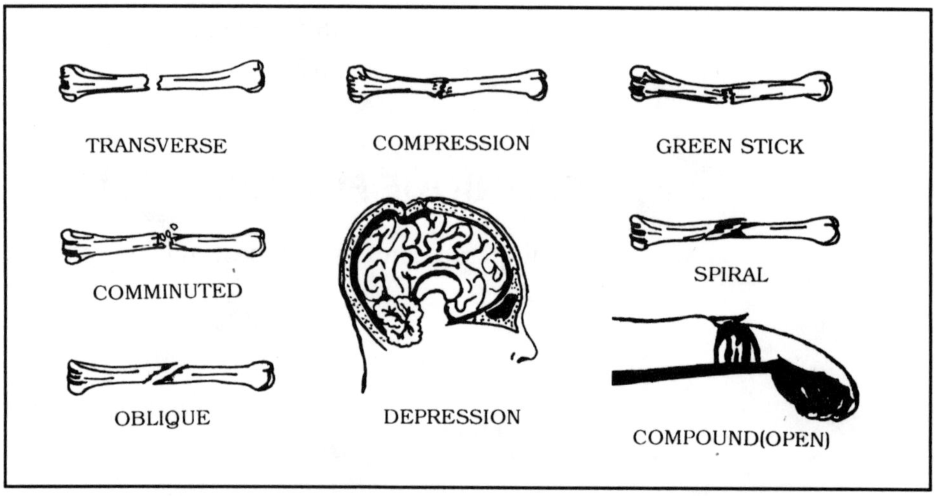

figure 5-3. Classification of fractures.

TECHNIQUE FOR TREATMENT:

1. Control any bleeding.
2. Prevent shock.
3. *CALL AN AMBULANCE*, or carefully splint possible fracture before transporting to emergency room. (If there is any doubt about severity, call paramedics.)

*Treatments continued on next page

4. You may apply ice to the possible fracture site to relieve pain and swelling. Take care to not displace possible fracture area.

SPLINTING

If you have any doubt concerning the extent of an injury, or you think someone has fractured a bone, you can completely immobilize the area by splinting before moving the athlete.

RULES FOR SPLINTING

1. Immobilize the injured area and the joints above and below the fracture.

2. If it is a compound fracture, *DO NOT ATTEMPT* to push the bone ends beneath the skin.

3. *DO NOT STRAIGHTEN EXTREMITY.* Splint it in its current position. Almost anything light and solid can be used for splinting: newspapers, pillows, hockey sticks, tongue depressors, etc. (Use your imagination if necessary.)

4. Keep victim as still as possible during movement and transport.

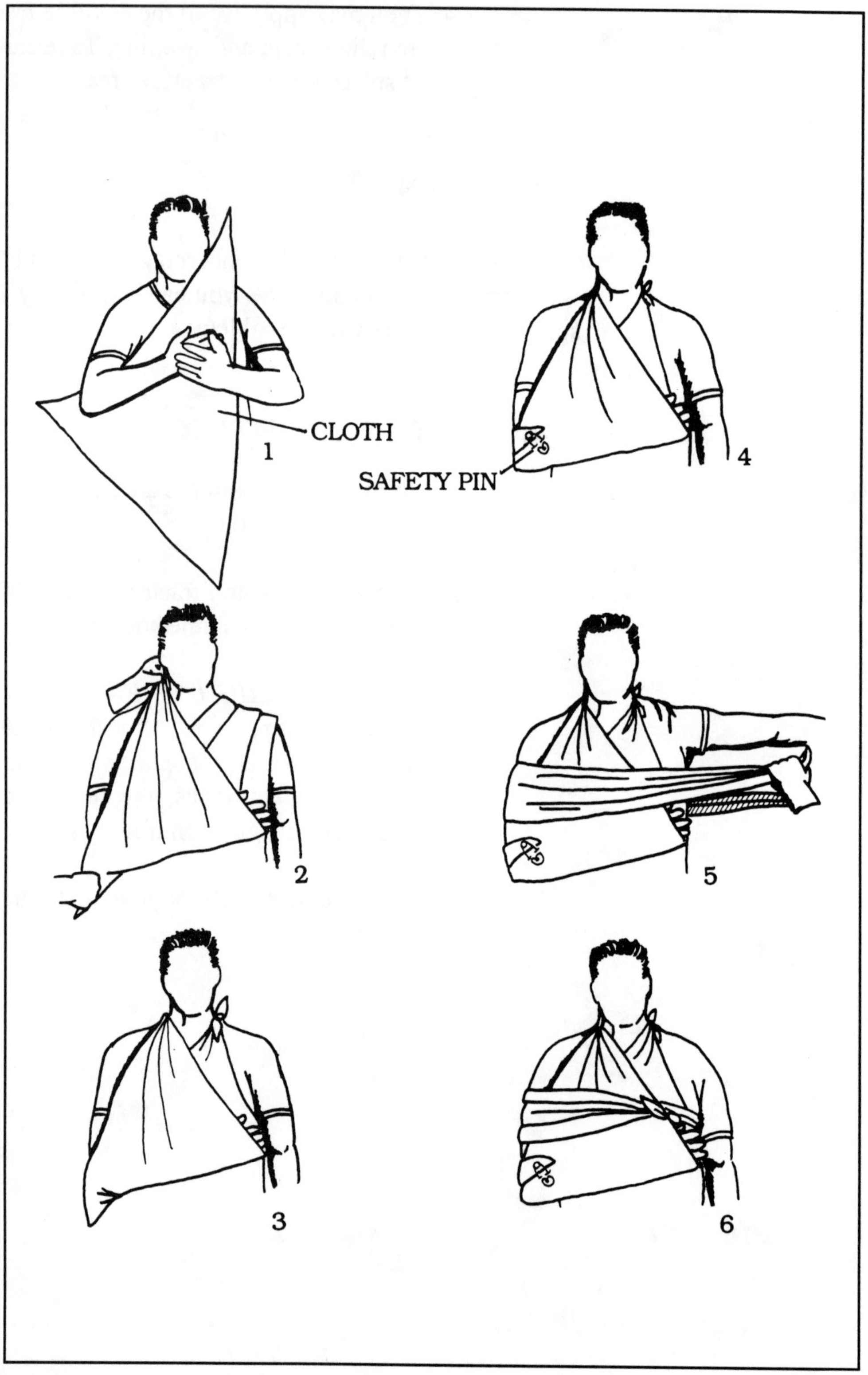

figure 5-4. Proper method of supporting the arm with a sling.

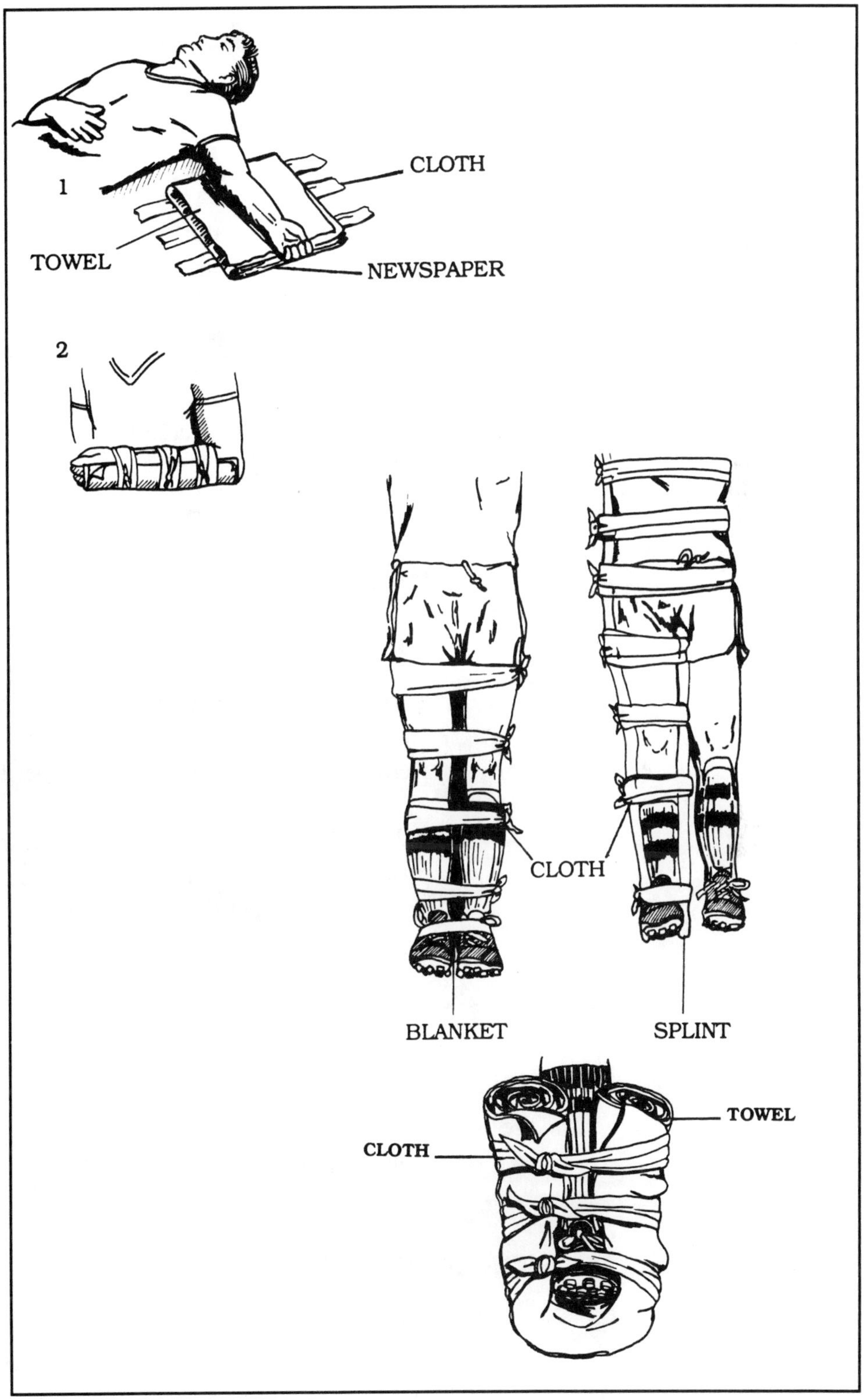

figure 5-5. Splinting techniques for the arm, leg, and ankle.

5.5 HEAT ILLNESS

HEAT CRAMPS

Improper fluid and mineral balance in the muscles due to loss of water, sodium, potassium and chlorine can cause heat cramps.

SIGNS/SYMPTOMS:

- Excessive sweating coupled with muscular spasm and cramping.

TECHNIQUE FOR TREATMENT:

1. Cool and shade victim.
2. Replenish water. Athlete should drink *slowly.*
3. Remove athlete from further competition.
4. Athlete should eat a proper diet that includes a proper sodium/chloride (salt), calcium and potassium content (see section 2.1).

HEAT EXHAUSTION

This condition occurs when blood is shunted to the capillaries in the skin to rid the body of excess heat. This leads to premature exhaustion because of the reduced circulation to the muscles, etc.

SIGNS/SYMPTOMS:

- Moist, clammy, usually pale skin
- Normal or subnormal body temperature

- •Excessive sweating
- •Dilated pupils
- •Fatigue, weakness, fainting due to heat
- •Nausea, dizziness.

TECHNIQUE FOR TREATMENT:

1. Remove or loosen clothing.

2. *COOL ATHLETE.* Remove from further competition. Fan and cool with wet towels, move to shade, etc. Do not chill athlete.

3. Athlete should lie down, elevate feet and relax.

4. Give water in very small amounts unless the athlete becomes nauseated or begins vomiting.

5. If the athlete does not recover quickly, take the person to emergency room.

figure 5-6. Signs and symptoms of heat exhaustion and heat stroke.

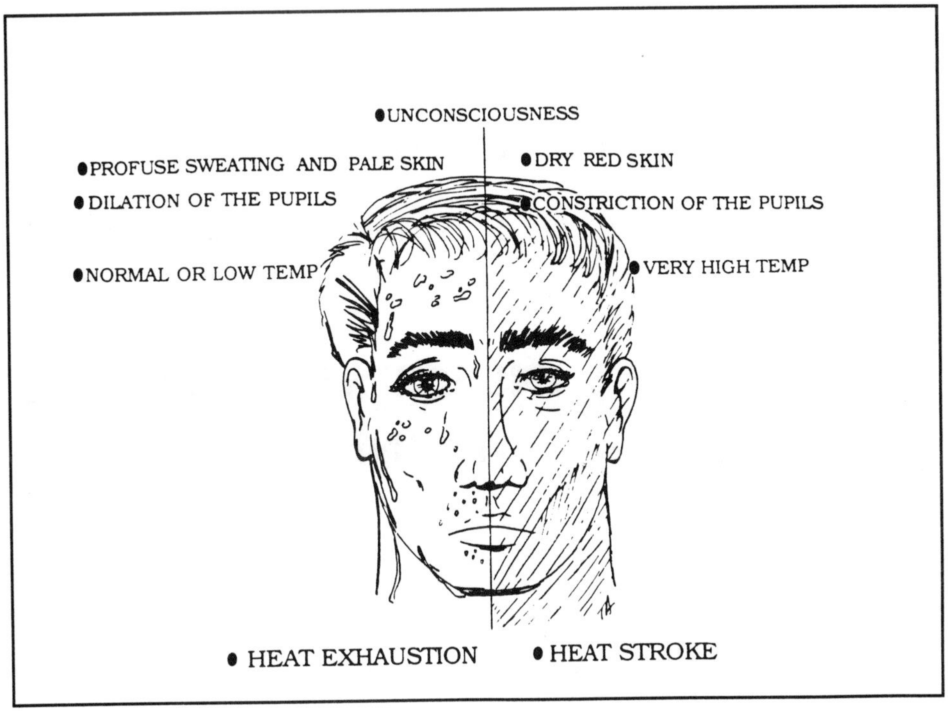

HEAT STROKE

Heat stroke is the failure of the body's heat regulating system. Use immediate first aid and call a paramedic.

** *LIFE THREATENING* ** *MEDICAL EMERGENCY* **

SIGNS/SYMPTOMS:

•Hot, dry, red skin
•Constricted pupils
•Extreme body temperatures
•Nausea, vomiting
•Rapid pulse and breathing
•Weak—may lose consciousness.

TECHNIQUE FOR TREATMENT:

** *TIME IS CRITICAL* **

1. Remove athlete from heat or sun.
2. Remove clothing.
3. Use ice, water, fanning or anything to cool athlete's body.
4. *CALL AN AMBULANCE IMMEDIATELY.*
5. *Do not* administer fluids.

5.6 INSECT STINGS AND OTHER POISONINGS

INSECT STINGS

** *Coaches should be aware of players who are allergic to bee stings.* **

If an athlete suffers sudden pain, and swelling occurred after an obvious or suspected insect sting, you may need to provide first aid.

SIGNS/SYMPTOMS:

- Swelling
- Localized pain
- Itching
- Red bump on skin associated with other symptoms.

TECHNIQUE FOR TREATMENT:

1. *WATCH FOR ALLERGIC REACTIONS:*
   - Excessive swelling, especially of face and tongue
   - Weakness or dizziness
   - Hives or excessive skin irritation
   - Spread of localized pain
   - Difficulty breathing
   - Chest or abdominal pain
   - Nausea, vomiting, cramps.

** *ANY ATHLETE WITH THESE SYMPTOMS SHOULD BE IMMEDIATELY TRANSPORTED TO AN EMERGENCY FACILITY.* **

2. You should have and use a bee sting kit *only* if an athlete is known *not* to react to the anti-venom. If an athlete has never used anti-venom, *DO NOT* use it because of the possibility of allergic reactions and possible infections.

3. To remove a visible stinger, use a fingernail or knife blade to scrape the stinger away from the wound.

4. Apply ice for swelling.

POISONING

If someone is found with pills, chemicals, etc., and is not feeling well, that person may have been poisoned. The victim may be conscious or unconscious.

SIGNS/SYMPTOMS:

•Sudden collapse
•Vomiting
•Labored breathing
•Excessive pupil dilation or constriction
•Victim cannot be aroused from a deep sleep
•Empty container nearby
•Burns around mouth area
•Victim's breath smells of gasoline, alcohol, etc.

TECHNIQUE FOR TREATMENT:

Conscious Victim

1. Try to identify the poison.

2. Contact poison control or emergency room.

3. While on the phone, *CONVEY THIS INFORMATION:*
   •What is wrong
   •Who you are
   •Where the victim is
   •Victim's age and condition
   •What poison was taken and how much (if known)
   •Any first aid you have already administered.

** DO NOT HANG UP THE PHONE.
LET THE POISON CONTROL CENTER HANG UP FIRST. **

** *If you are unable to make contact, give one glassful of milk or water for an adult. Give less for a child.* **

*Treatment continued on the next page.

4. Treat for shock.

Unconscious Victim

1. Check ABCs (see section 6.1).
2. *DO NOT* give the victim anything to eat or drink.
3. Try to identify the poison.
4. *Contact the poison control center or emergency room as soon as possible.*
5. Place the victim on one side so fluids such as vomit will flow out of the mouth and not block the airway.

5.7 LIGAMENTOUS INJURIES

An injury to a ligament caused by hyperextension, dislocation, subluxation or excessive twisting or rotation of a joint is called a **sprain**. Sprains are defined according to their severity: first degree, second degree and third degree.

FIRST DEGREE SPRAIN

A minor stretching or twisting of a ligament is called a first degree sprain.

SIGNS/SYMPTOMS:

- Swelling
- Minor pain when touched and moved
- Slight loosening of ligament.

TECHNIQUE FOR TREATMENT:

1. Apply R-I-C-E treatment (p. 164).

2. Continue to use proper cold therapy treatments until trauma has subsided (p. 164).

SECOND DEGREE SPRAIN

A moderate twist, pull or partial tear of a ligament that produces a slight looseness of the joint is called a second degree sprain.

SIGNS/SYMPTOMS:

•Swelling, skin discoloration
•Pain upon movement
•Slight looseness of joint.

TECHNIQUE FOR TREATMENT:

1. *DO NOT* let athlete walk off field if the injury is in the hips, knees or ankles.

2. Apply R-I-C-E treatment (p. 164).

3. Withdraw athlete from further competition that day.

4. Isolate joint from unnecessary movement.

5. Refer to physician for proper examination.

** *SEVERE SPRAINS MAY BE ASSOCIATED WITH A FRACTURE.* **

THIRD DEGREE SPRAIN

A major twist or pull on the ligament that causes a severe or complete tear is called a third degree sprain.

SIGNS/SYMPTOMS:

- •Loss of proper joint function
- •Extreme pain
- •Swelling, skin discoloration
- •Obvious looseness, possible joint deformity
- •Extreme tenderness.

TECHNIQUE FOR TREATMENT:

1. The joint should be completely immobilized before moving and transporting (see p. 109).

2. Apply R-I-C-E treatment as soon as possible (p. 164).

3. Seek medical attention.

figure 5-7. Various degrees of SPRAIN of the lateral collateral ligament (knee).

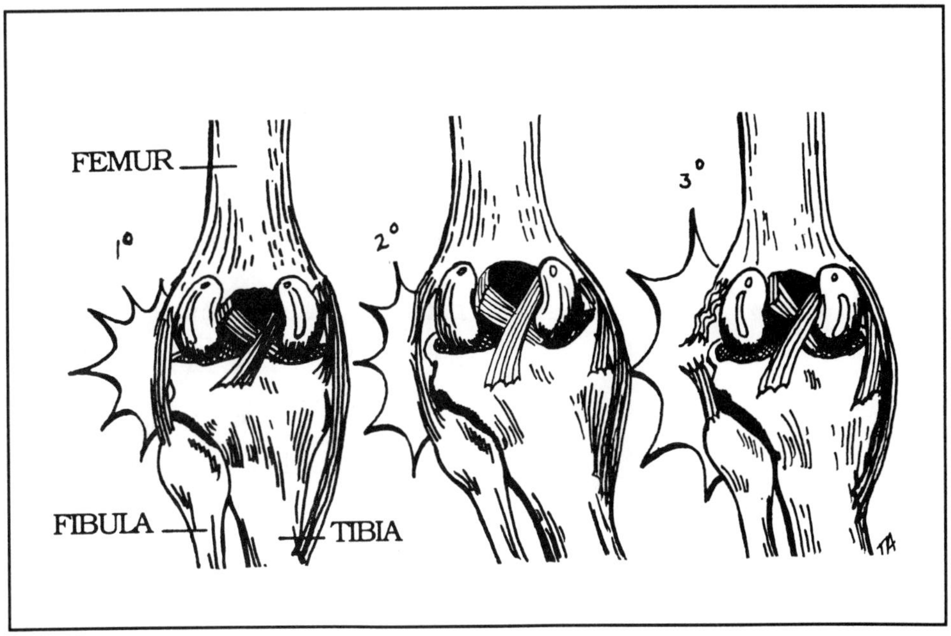

5.8 MUSCULAR-TENDINOUS INJURIES

Any pulling or tearing of a muscle or tendon is called a **strain**. Like sprains, strains are divided into groups according to the severity of the injury: first degree, second degree and third degree. Strains are usually caused by overextension (stretching) or a forced movement of a muscle, which causes ripping or straining.

FIRST DEGREE STRAIN

A first degree strain indicates as slight muscle overstretch or excessive forced contraction.

SIGNS/SYMPTOMS:

•Soreness in muscle
•Slight tenderness to touch
•Slight muscular spasm.

TECHNIQUE FOR TREATMENT:

1. Apply R-I-C-E treatment (p. 164).

2. Follow with very mild, comfortable stretching of muscle.

3. The athlete may return to activity if the muscle is supported and there is no pain or loss of strength.

4. If athlete is not well enough to return to activity, continue to use cold therapy technique (p. 164).

5. *Do not* apply heat for at least 48 hours or until all swelling and initial trauma has subsided.

6. Athlete should constantly stretch the muscle mildly every chance possible.

*Treatments continued on next page

7. Follow with proper heat treatments and stretching exercises (p. 165, 73) for rehabilitation.

8. Be sure the athlete has regained full strength and range of motion before allowing a return to competition.

SECOND DEGREE STRAIN

A second degree strain is a moderate overstretching of muscle and includes slight tearing of muscle fibers.

SIGNS/SYMPTOMS:

- Swelling
- Tenderness when touched and moved
- Initial sharp pain at injury site
- Muscle spasms
- Partial loss of muscle function or range of motion.

TECHNIQUE FOR TREATMENT:

1. Apply R-I-C-E treatment (p. 164).

2. Withdraw athlete from further competition that day.

3. Isolate movement of injured muscle as much as possible by applying flexible bandage wrap or sling, and using crutches if necessary.

4. Have a sports injury professional evaluate the injury for proper rehabilitation.

THIRD DEGREE STRAIN

A third degree strain indicates a moderate to complete tear of muscle by excessive muscle stretch or contraction.

SIGNS/SYMPTOMS:

- •Extreme pain
- •Loss of muscle function
- •A snap or pop
- •Swelling
- •Skin discoloration
- •Muscular spasms
- •Extreme tenderness.

TECHNIQUE FOR TREATMENT:

1. Same techniques as for second degree strains, but make sure the muscle is completely immobilized.

2. Have a physician check the injury for further treatment.

figure 5-8. Various degrees of STRAIN of the biceps femoris (hamstring) muscle.

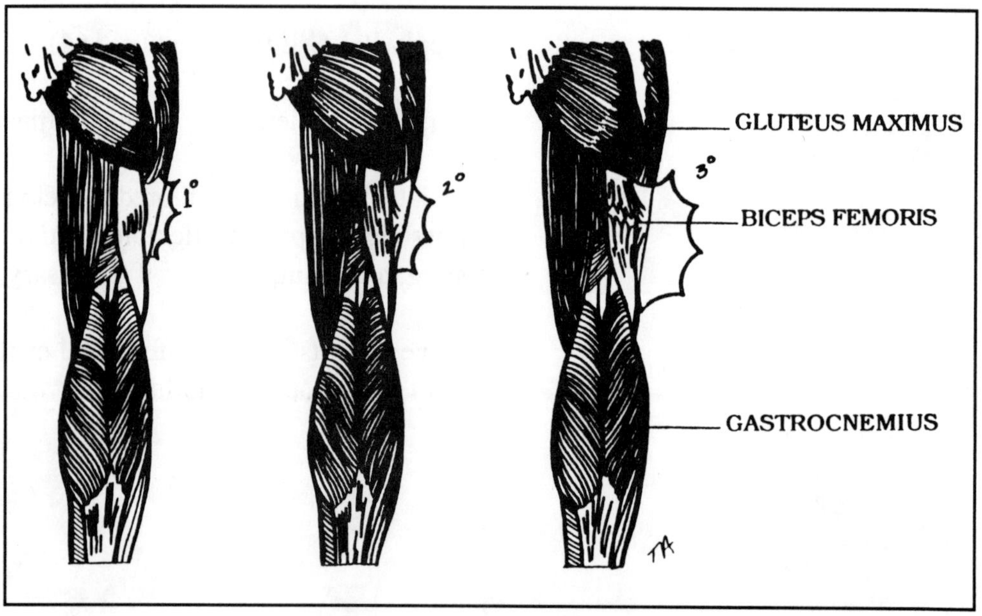

MYOSITIS OSSIFICANS (CALCIUM DEPOSITS IN MUSCLE TISSUE)

In this condition, the natural body process of healing is not allowed to continue because the muscle did not heal properly before returning to competition, or the muscle is chronically bruised by repeated injury. Instead of normal scar tissue replacement, calcium builds up in the muscle, which ossifies, or turns to bone.

SIGNS/SYMPTOMS:

•Hard, painful places can be felt when palpating muscle
•Chronic muscle pain in area.

PREVENTIVE TREATMENT:

1. Make sure all muscle injuries are properly healed. Full range of motion, strength and painless movement must be regained before an athlete should return to competition.

2. To prevent chronic re-injury, use protective padding or provide proper support for muscle group.

TECHNIQUE FOR TREATMENT:

If you suspect an athlete may have calcium deposits, withdraw that person from further competition and refer him or her to an orthopedic surgeon for examination.

TENDINITIS (TENNIS ELBOW, ETC.)

Inflammation of tendons due to too much stress is called tendinitis.

SIGNS/SYMPTOMS:

•Pain
•Swelling
•Grating feeling during movement of tendon
•Limited joint movement.

TECHNIQUE FOR TREATMENT:

1. Apply ice therapy (p. 164).

2. Discontinue training and competition until symptoms disappear.

3. Stretch area two or three times per day.

4. Thoroughly warm up area before restarting training. Analgesic balms and supportive wraps may help decrease the discomfort.

5. If conditions persist for more than four days without training, consult a physician.

5.9 SEIZURES

A seizure is any attack triggered by epilepsy, illness or a sharp blow to the head. Two basic types of seizures are **grand mal** and **petit mal**.

SIGNS/SYMPTOMS:

Grand Mal

•Convulsions
•Loss of consciousness
•Breathing stopped.

Petit mal

•Dazed. Petit mal seizures are actually often undetected.

TECHNIQUE FOR TREATMENT:

1. Catch or *gently* lower the victim to the ground.
2. Keep the victim from harm as much as possible, but *DO NOT* restrain the victim.
3. Loosen tight clothing, uniform, etc.
4. *DO NOT* place any object or fingers into the victim's mouth.
5. *CALL AN AMBULANCE.*
6. If possible, place the victim on his or her side to let secretions flow from the mouth.
7. *Note for the paramedics the LENGTH and TIME of the seizure.*

5.10 SHOCK

Shock occurs when not enough blood is circulated throughout the body. It is caused by cardiovascular failure or any sudden trauma to the body, such as a severe injury, excessive blood loss, respiratory obstruction or allergic reaction. Shock depresses normal body functions and can keep organs and muscles from working normally because of the lack of consistent blood pressure.

** CAN BE LIFE-THREATENING **

** *GIVE IMMEDIATE FIRST AID AND CALL THE PARAMEDICS* **

SIGNS/SYMPTOMS:

•Shallow, rapid breathing
•Rapid, weak pulse
•Pale, clammy skin
•Shaking, trembling, sweating
•Enlarged pupils
•Dizziness, tiredness (weakness)
•Nausea, vomiting.

TECHNIQUE FOR TREATMENT:

1. Check ABCs. (see section 6.1)

2. Control bleeding with gentle compression (see p. 103).

3. Reassure, quiet and soothe victim.

4. Maintain normal body temperature. If it is hot, shade the victim. If it is cool, warm the victim.

5. If the lower body is injured, elevate the legs 12 inches, unless serious injury is suspected.

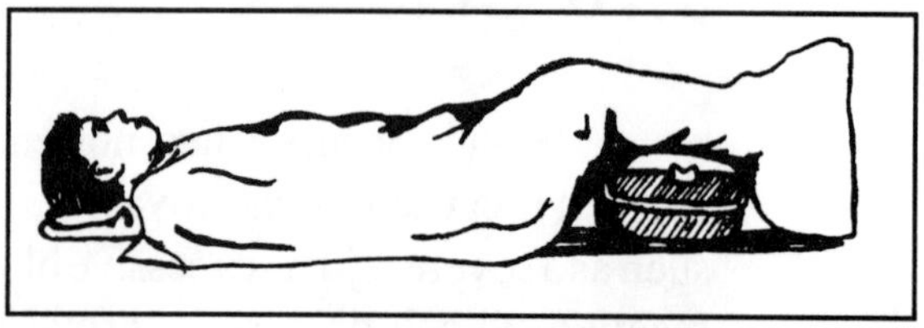

6. If the head or chest is injured, elevate the upper body, unless serious injury is suspected.

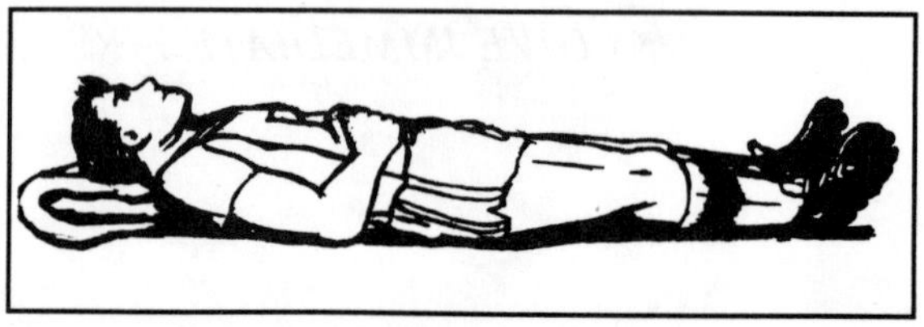

*Treatment continued on next page

7. If unsure as to what to elevate or if serious injury is suspected, leave victim flat on the ground.

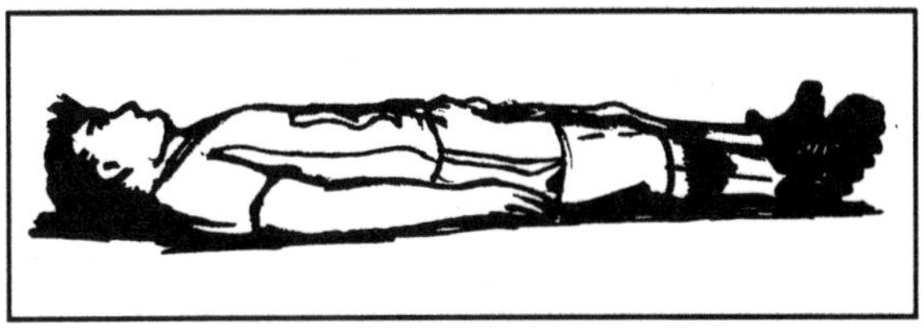

8. Do not administer fluids or foods unless medical care will be delayed.

9. Call an ambulance.

5.11 WOUNDS

This section covers four types of wounds: abrasions, blisters, closed and open wounds.

** *Always wear surgical gloves when dealing with open wounds to protect against diseases that can be transmitted by blood, such as AIDS and hepatitis.* **

ABRASIONS

If only the top layer of skin is scraped off leaving pink tissue below, it is called an abrasion. On the field an abrasion is often called a "strawberry."

SIGNS/SYMPTOMS:

•Bleeding
•Oozing

- Pain
- Pink, fleshy tissue is visible because of the removal of the top layer of skin.

TECHNIQUE FOR TREATMENT:

1. Treat as an open wound.

2. Keep wound moist with a first aid cream, but do not cover. This can help prevent a chronic injury.

BLISTERS

A blister occurs when layers of skin are separated because of abnormal shearing forces or friction on the skin.

SIGNS/SYMPTOMS:

- Torn layer of skin
- Water-like bubble under skin
- Oozing
- Red or painful place on skin.

TECHNIQUE FOR TREATMENT:

1. If the blister has broken, treat as an open wound. If skin is not broken, DO NOT puncture blister and proceed to step 3.

2. Clean with soap and water, and apply ointment with a protective dressing.

3. If painful, use felt or moleskin to remove the pressure from the sore area.

CLOSED WOUNDS
(CONTUSIONS, HEMATOMAS)

A bruising of tissue caused by a blunt object striking the body surface is called a closed wound, or a contusion. If blood visibly pools under the skin from internal bleeding and a blood blister develops, the injury is called a hematoma.

SIGNS/SYMPTOMS:

•Blue/red skin discoloration caused by internal bleeding
•Dark colored blister
•Swelling
•Partial loss of muscle function at injury site
•Pain.

TECHNIQUE FOR TREATMENT:

1. Apply R-I-C-E treatment (p. 164)

2. If contusion is on the head, neck or spine, evaluate injury first.

3. If underlying fracture is suspected, treat accordingly (p. 107).

4. *DO NOT* allow athlete to participate until the contusion is healed to avoid calcium development in the muscle tissue (p. 123).

OPEN WOUNDS (PUNCTURES, INCISIONS, AVULSIONS, LACERATIONS)

A cut or slice through the skin is called an open wound. It can be caused by impalement.

SIGNS/SYMPTOMS:

- •Open cut or puncture wound
- •Bleeding
- •Pain.

TECHNIQUE FOR TREATMENT:

1. Fully expose wound when possible. Cut away clothing, tape, etc., only if necessary.

2. Control bleeding (see p. 103).

3. Remove foreign matter from the surface of the wound.

4. Treat to prevent shock.

5. If wound is not serious (deep) and bleeding is completely controlled, cleanse wound with a topical hydrogen peroxide solution or by blotting with a mild soap and towel. *Do not rub.* Cover with a sterile bandage. If athlete returns to competition, the bandaging can be secured by applying tincture of benzoin to the wound and the area around it. This tincture becomes tacky when dry and helps the bandages stick to the skin. Continue to monitor victim for shock.

figure 5-9. Classification of open wounds.

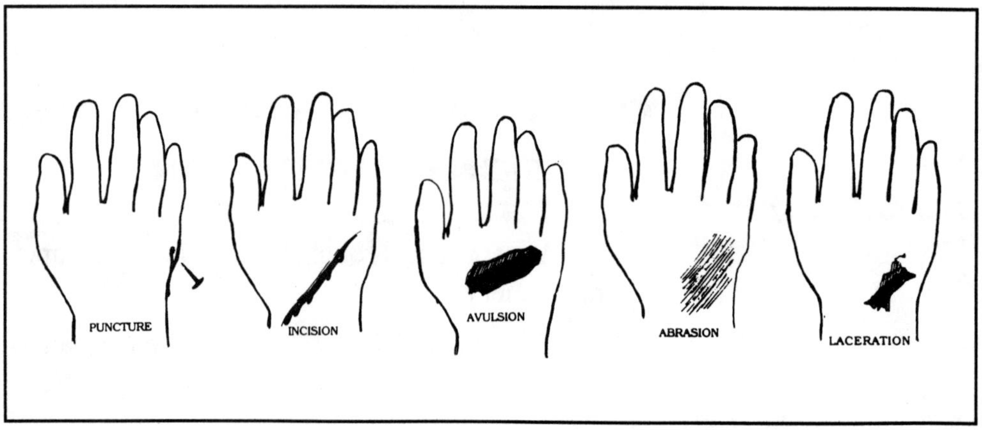

6 Recognition and Care of Specific Injuries

While the last chapter covered conditions that affect the whole body or could occur anywhere in the body, this chapter addresses specific injuries and conditions.

6.1 GENERAL INJURY PROCEDURE

Even if an injury is obvious, you must make certain no other problems threaten. By following certain rules and steps, you can not only properly evaluate athletic injuries, you can also prevent further injury.

Follow these steps whenever possible, necessary and appropriate:

1. Check for consciousness. If the person is conscious, reassure and calm the athlete.

2. Check ABCs.
   A = **airway**. Ensure the airway passage from the mouth to the lungs.
   B = look, listen and feel for **breathing**. If the victim is not breathing, start mouth-to-mouth resuscitation.
   C = check the pulse for **circulation**. If there is no pulse, begin CPR.

3. Control bleeding.

4. Expose the injured area by removing clothing, socks, shoelaces, shoes, etc.

5. Determine what structures are involved. Ask the athlete:
   •*How* it happened
   •*Where* it hurts
   •*What* the other athletes and/or observers *saw, heard, or felt.*

6. *CHECK THE ENTIRE BODY*, head to toe, visually and by palpation for pain, deformity, swelling, lack of movement,

abnormal skin color and condition, reaction of the eye pupils to light, shock symptoms, medical alert tags, etc.

7. Administer proper first aid, according to the injury or problem.

8. Treat athlete mentally as well as physically.

9. Get proper medical attention when needed.

table 6-1. Protocol for quick examination of an injured athlete. Start with primary survey and continue with secondary survey if appropriate.

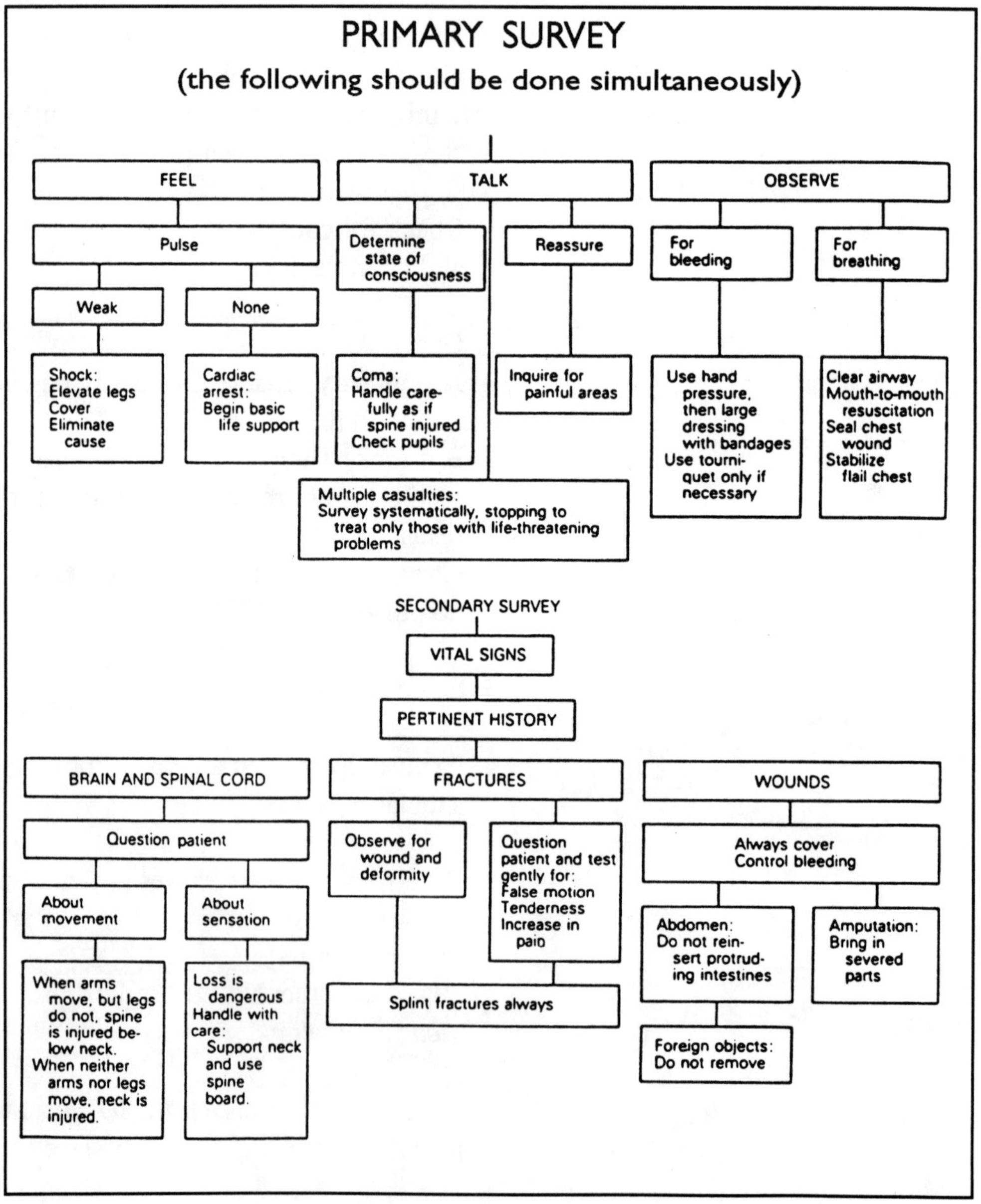

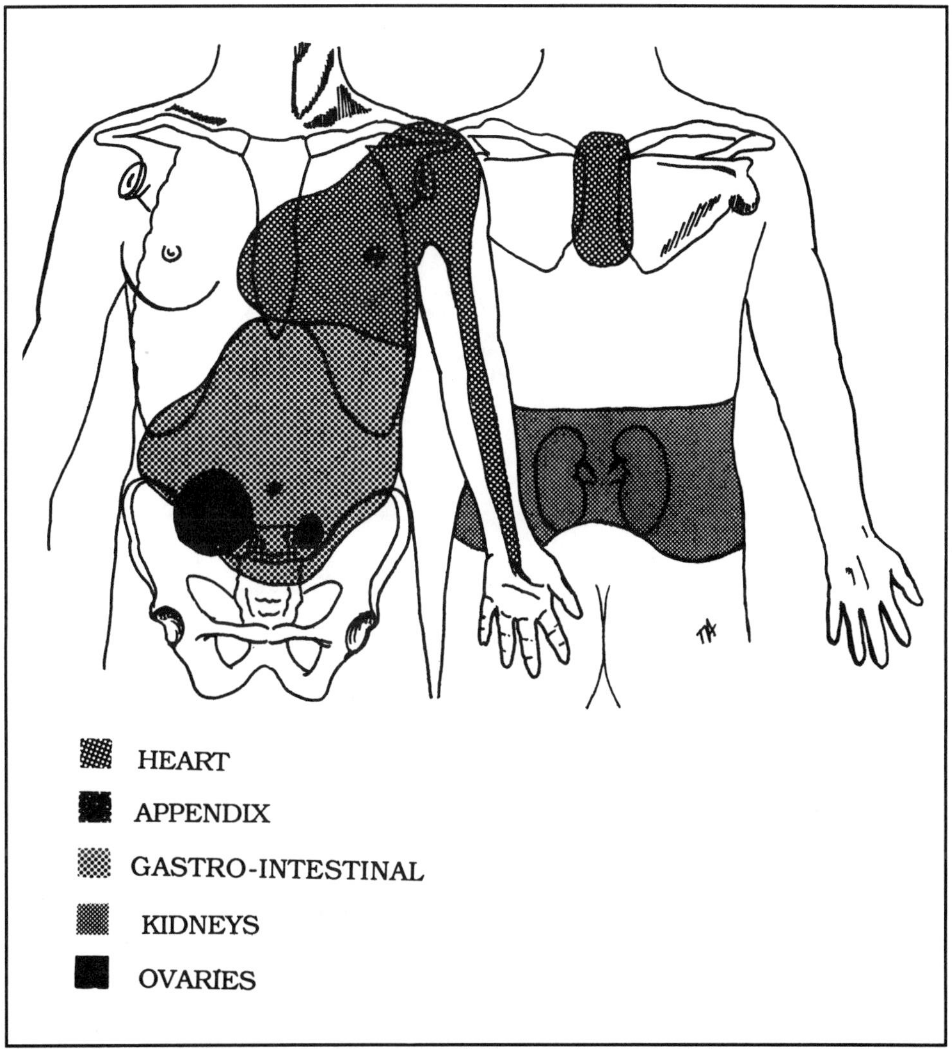

figure 6-1. Pain in certain body parts is often associated with specific injuries and illnesses. A few of these common regions, with the associated organs, are shown here.

6.2 HEAD INJURIES

figure 6-2. Bony anatomy of the head.

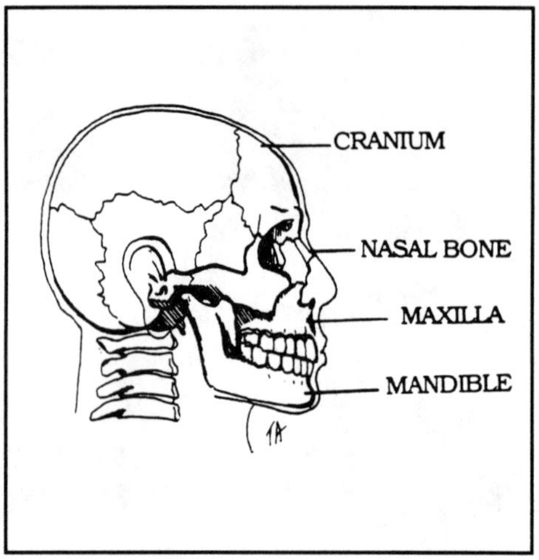

MECHANISM OF INJURY:

Any force to the head by collision or contact from a foreign body. Injuries can be minor to permanently disabling. Open head wounds usually bleed considerably.

SIGNS/SYMPTOMS:

•* Unequal pupils
•* Loss of consciousness
•* Deformity of skull
•* Bleeding from ears or nose
•* Clear fluids coming from ears, nose, mouth
•Open wound, bleeding from wound
•Tenderness, swelling
•Facial muscles partially paralyzed or not working properly
•Nausea or vomiting
•Loss of balance, dizziness.

TECHNIQUE FOR TREATMENT:

1. Check ABCs. (see section 6.1)

2. If any of the starred (*) items above are present, *DO NOT* move athlete, and *CALL AN AMBULANCE IMMEDIATELY.*

*Treatment continued on next page.

3. Control bleeding from wounds, but *DO NOT stop bleeding and fluid flow from ears and nose.*

4. If this is a serious injury, immobilize the victim's head, neck and spine.

5. For minor bruises and bumps on the head, apply ice.

6. If the athlete is continuously conscious and otherwise feels perfectly fine, administer the **Romberg Test**: Have the athlete stand straight with arms at sides, feet together and eyes closed. If the victim is unable to maintain balance, this is a sign of a neuro-cranial disturbance, and you should refer the athlete to medical care.

7. *If you are in doubt about the athlete's condition, ALWAYS remove the athlete from further competition.*

*** IF AN ATHLETE LOSES CONSCIOUSNESS FOR ANY REASON, THE INDIVIDUAL SHOULD NOT RETURN TO THE ACTIVITY. ***

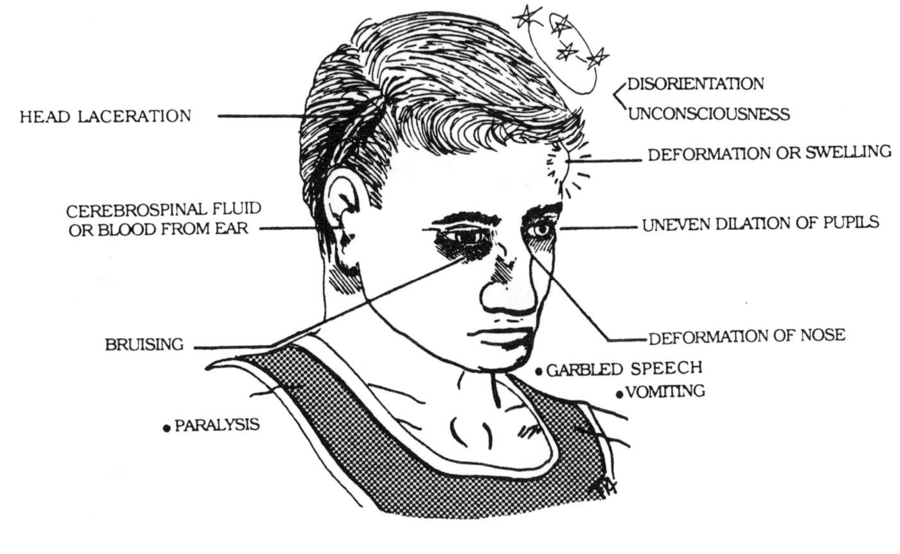

figure 6-3. Common signs and symptoms of head injuries.

*** CONSTANTLY MONITOR anyone with a head injury for delayed symptoms. Symptoms often are not noticeable at first and will develop later. DO NOT administer any aspirin or other drugs that may mask the delayed symptoms. Keep liquid intake to a minimum. ***

DELAYED SIGNS/SYMPTOMS:

- Severe headache
- Persistent vomiting
- Unequal pupil size
- Slurred speech
- Blurry or double vision
- Excessive tiredness or drowsiness.

*** Parents should monitor the victim for 24 hours after the trauma, waking the athlete periodically to check for delayed signs/symptoms. ***

6.3 NECK AND SPINE INJURIES

MECHANISM OF INJURY:

A sharp blow, twist or any excessive bending of the neck and spine. Can cause permanent paralysis.

SIGNS/SYMPTOMS:

- Pain in neck or spine area with or without movement
- Loss of feeling or a prickling sensation in the extremities
- Loss of grip strength or unequal grip strength in hands
- Tenderness
- Deformity of neck or spinal area
- Wounds
- Breathing difficulty.

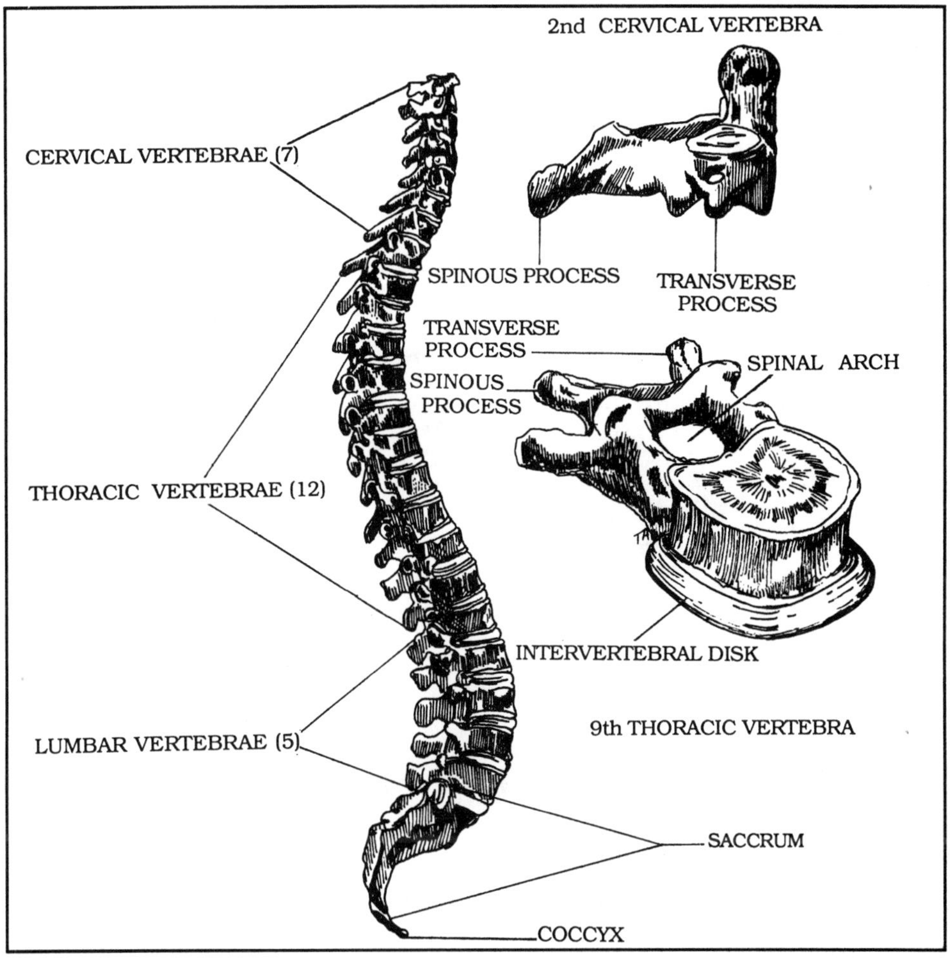

figure 6-4. Bony anatomy of the neck and spine.

TECHNIQUE FOR TREATMENT:

1. If the injury occurs while playing sports that require helmets, *DO NOT REMOVE A PLAYER'S HELMET UNLESS IT IS NECESSARY TO SAVE THE ATHLETE'S LIFE.*

2. *DO NOT MOVE THE ATHLETE FROM THE ORIGINAL POSITION.*

3. *CALL AMBULANCE.*

*Treatment continued on next page.

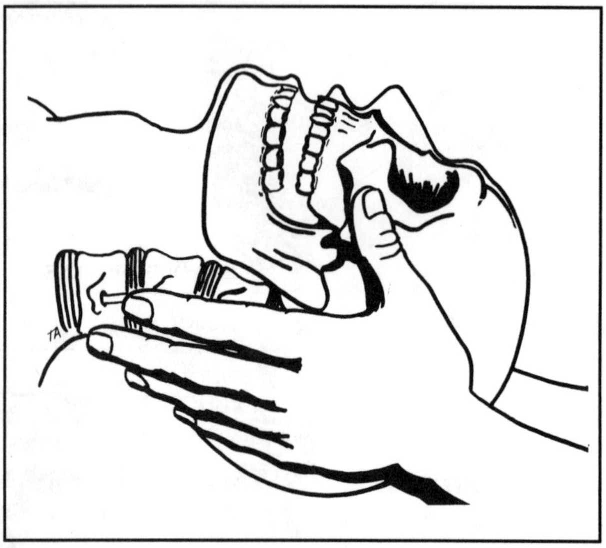

figure 6-5. Technique for isolation of the neck. Use caution not to move the neck when placing hands in position.

4. *ISOLATE THE VICTIM'S NECK AND SPINE FROM ANY MOVEMENT IF POSSIBLE WITHOUT MOVING ATHLETE (figure 6-5).*

5. Treat for shock.

6. Constantly check the victim's ABCs.

7. Constantly reassure and talk with the athlete until medical help arrives.

6.4 FACE INJURIES

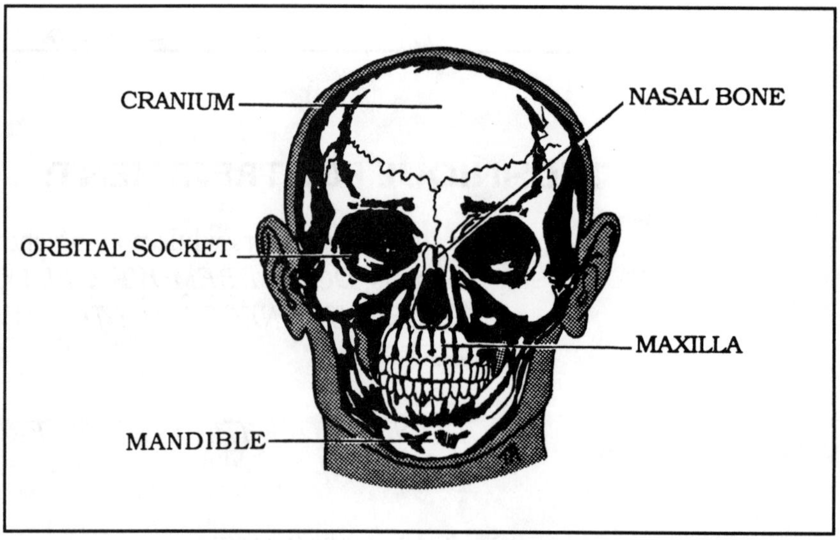

figure 6-6. Bony anatomy of the face.

MECHANISM OF INJURY:

Any blow to the eyes, nose, teeth or maxillo-facial area.

EYES

TECHNIQUE FOR EMERGENCY CARE:

1. Wash the eye *only* in the event of chemical injury.
2. If the eyeball has been perforated, *DO NOT wash.* Put a loose dressing over both eyes and *transport immediately to the emergency room.*
3. Because both eyes move together, after any serious blow to the eye *cover both eyes* to limit movement.
4. Be aware of possible head injuries.

Detached Retina

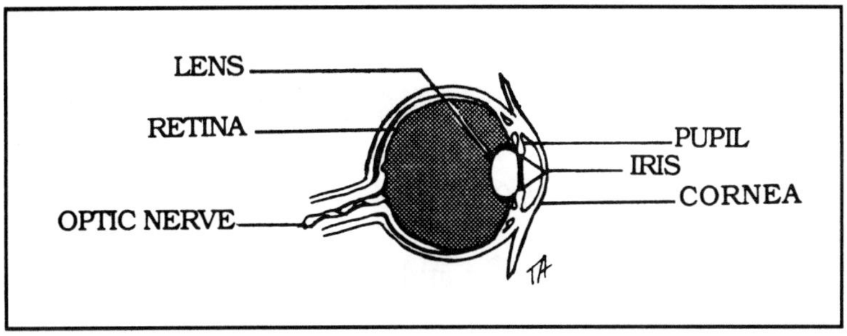

SIGNS/SYMPTOMS:

•Light flashes in vision
•Dark spots or "curtain" blocking vision.

TECHNIQUE FOR TREATMENT:

1. *CALL AN AMBULANCE. The athlete must be transported very carefully.*

2. Keep the athlete still, preferably lying on his or her back.

** *REALIZE THAT THE INJURY MAY BE CAUSED BY BLOW TO THE HEAD, NOT JUST THE EYE, AND TREAT ACCORDINGLY.* **

Orbital Socket Fractures

SIGNS/SYMPTOMS:

•Swelling and tenderness around the eyes
•Blue/black skin discoloration around an eye
•Numbness around eye
•Double or blurred vision
•Partial loss of the visual field.

TECHNIQUE FOR TREATMENT:

1. *CALL AN AMBULANCE IMMEDIATELY.*

2. If desired, apply ice to reduce swelling.

3. Cover *both* eyes to prevent movement of eyeballs.

4. Keep athlete sitting and calm.

Removing Foreign Matter From the Eye

TECHNIQUE FOR TREATMENT:

1. Try to make athlete produce tears by blinking.

2. *DO NOT RUB THE EYE.*

3. If the item is not removed by tear flow, wash your hands if possible and have the athlete look upward. Carefully pull out bottom eyelid and examine for foreign matter. If there is no material visible, repeat procedure with upper lid. To pull up the upper eyelid, place your thumb over upper lid and eyelash and push directly up. Use a soft, clean cloth to remove the material. *Never use dry cotton around the eye.*

Torn or Cut Eyelids

SIGNS/SYMPTOMS:

•Bleeding of eyelid
•Obvious tear on eyelid
•Cut on eyelid.

TECHNIQUE FOR TREATMENT:

** *TIME IS CRITICAL. BLINDNESS WILL RESULT IF EYELID IS NOT REPLACED AND THE EYE IS NOT KEPT MOIST.* **

1. If the eyelid is completely severed from body, wrap it in very moist towels and *transport the athlete and eyelid to the hospital immediately.*

2. If the eyelid is still attached, cover it with loose and moist dressing, cover both eyes and transport to the hospital.

*Treatment continued on next page.

3. Apply direct pressure to control bleeding. If the eyeball is also cut, *do not* apply pressure. Use loose bandaging and transport to *emergency room. HANDLE VERY CAREFULLY*

NOSE

Nose Bleeds

MECHANISM OF INJURY:

Any blow to the nose, physical stress, high blood pressure or infection can trigger nose bleeds. These injuries usually are not serious if bleeding is controlled quickly.

SIGNS/SYMPTOMS:

•Bleeding
•Swelling
•Pain.

TECHNIQUE FOR TREATMENT:

1. Have athlete sit up and lean forward.

2. Apply direct pressure by pinching the nostrils with the fingers.

3. Apply ice to nose area.

4. If bleeding continues, insert cotton or gauze into nostril and apply pressure.

5. If the nose bleeds more than 15 minutes, seek medical care.

Nose Fractures

SIGNS/SYMPTOMS:

•Deformity
•Blue/black skin discoloration
•Swelling
•Pain
•Bleeding.

TECHNIQUE FOR TREATMENT:

1. Control bleeding.
2. Apply ice.
3. Transport to emergency.

TEETH

MECHANISM OF INJURY:

Blow to the mouth where a tooth is knocked out or badly chipped.

SIGNS/SYMPTOMS:

•Tooth missing
•Pain
•Bleeding.

TECHNIQUE FOR TREATMENT:

1. If the tooth has come out of the socket, place it back into the socket if possible, or place it in a cup of water or wrap it in a moist cloth.
2. If the tooth is broken off rather than knocked out, cover the exposed pulp with a moist cloth or towel.

*Treatment continued on next page.

3. Transport the victim to a dentist or emergency room as soon as possible to try to save the tooth.

** *Athletes should use properly fitted mouthpieces to reduce dental trauma. Mouthpieces absorb shock from blows to the jaw, which can also decrease the possibility of a concussion.* **

6.5 CHEST INJURIES

MECHANISM OF INJURY:

Any sharp or blunt blow to the chest that damages the internal structures of the chest area above the diaphragm. Injuries may be open (visible) or closed (internal).

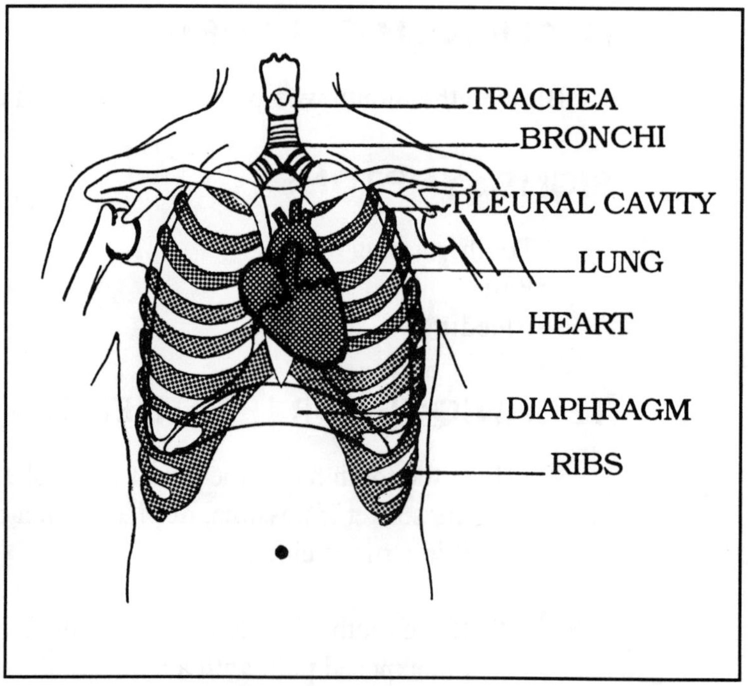

figure 6-7. Anatomy of the chest cavity.

SIGNS/SYMPTOMS:

•Tenderness, pain in chest area
•Obvious wound
•Painful or difficult breathing
•Bluish skin discoloration
•Nausea or vomiting
•Coughing up blood.

SIGNS/SYMPTOMS OF *HEART ATTACK:*

•Weakness
•Nausea
•Pain that travels to the shoulders, arms and neck
•Pressure, fullness or squeezing in chest area
•Feeling of indigestion accompanied with other symptoms
•Sharp chest pain
•Pain radiating down left arm
•Shortness of breath.

SIGNS/SYMPTOMS OF *LUNG DAMAGE:*

•Puncture wound in chest
•Wheezing, whistling sound coming through wound
•Inability to breath deeply.

SIGNS/SYMPTOMS OF *RIB FRACTURE:*

•Rib cage deformity
•Pain in rib area
•Pain from deep breathing
•Coughing.

TECHNIQUES FOR TREATMENT:

1. Check and maintain ABCs. (see section 6.1)

2. Treat for shock.

3. If the injury is localized and is accompanied with severe pain, deformity, loss of consciousness, swelling or bleeding, *DO NOT* move athlete; *CALL AN AMBULANCE.*

4. *DO NOT GIVE FOOD OR DRINK.*

figure 6-8. Signs and symptoms of chest injuries.

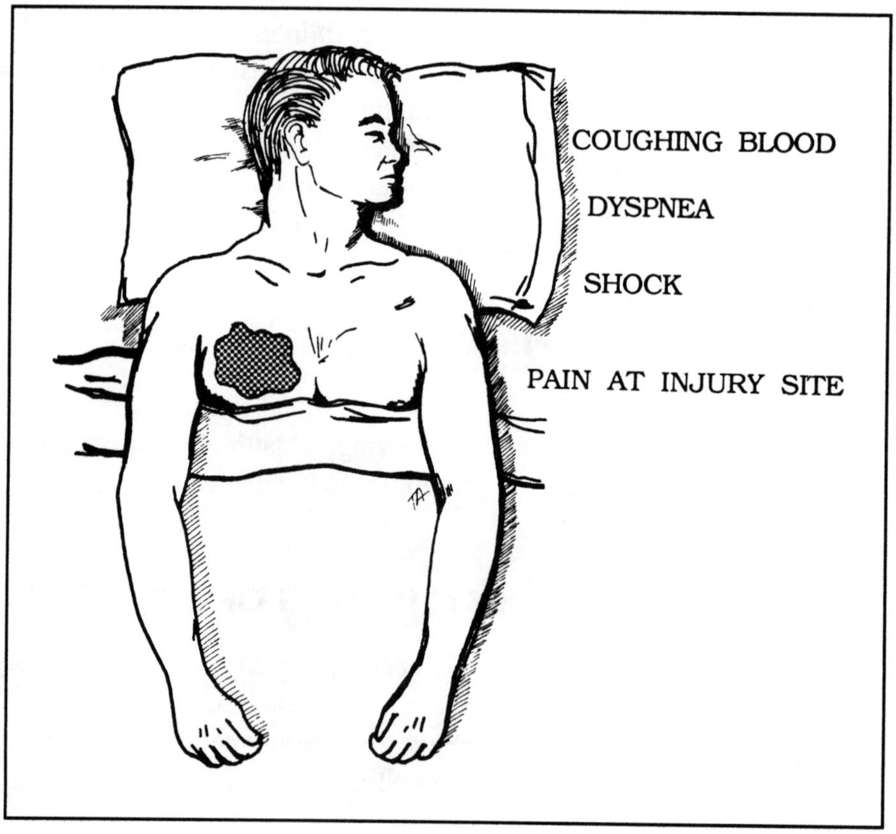

6.6 ABDOMINAL INJURIES

MECHANISM OF INJURY:

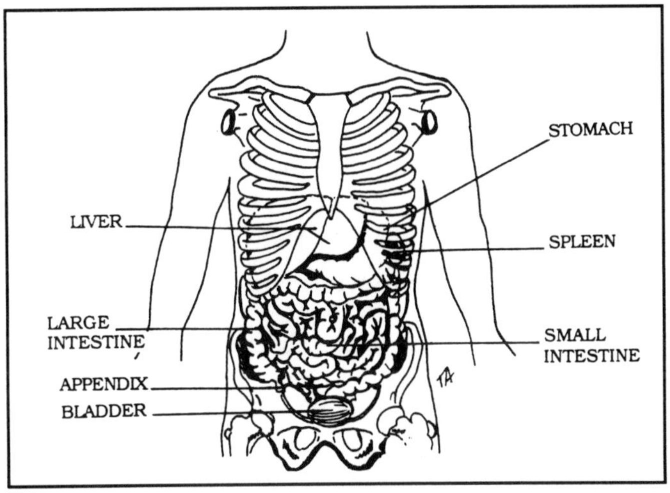

figure 6-9. Major organs in the abdomen.

Sharp or blunt blow to the anterior or posterior abdomen. Injuries range from minor to life threatening. The organs most susceptible to injury are the spleen, liver and kidneys.

SIGNS/SYMTOMS:

- Rapid, weak pulse
- Nausea
- Clammy skin
- Faintness
- Rock-hard abdomen, tense abdominal muscles
- Tenderness, swelling, pain
- Obvious wounds
- Protruded abdomen (which usually indicates internal bleeding)
- Victim draws up legs to alleviate pain
- Pain that appears, subsides and then reappears
- Pain in the left shoulder area (indicates a possible ruptured spleen).

** *IF ANY OF THESE SYMPTOMS ARE PRESENT, CALL AN AMBULANCE IMMEDIATELY.* **

TECHNIQUE FOR TREATMENT:

1. *DO NOT move athlete.*
2. Prevent shock.
3. *DO NOT give the victim anything to eat or drink.*
4. If the athlete feels OK after injury, monitor him or her carefully for the rest of the day and inform parents or guardians of the injury and the need to remain vigilant.
5. Victims who feel intense pain in the abdominal muscles can draw up their legs to alleviate pain.
6. If medical help will be delayed, palpate each of the four abdominal quadrants and note any abnormalities. Then call the emergency room for further directions.

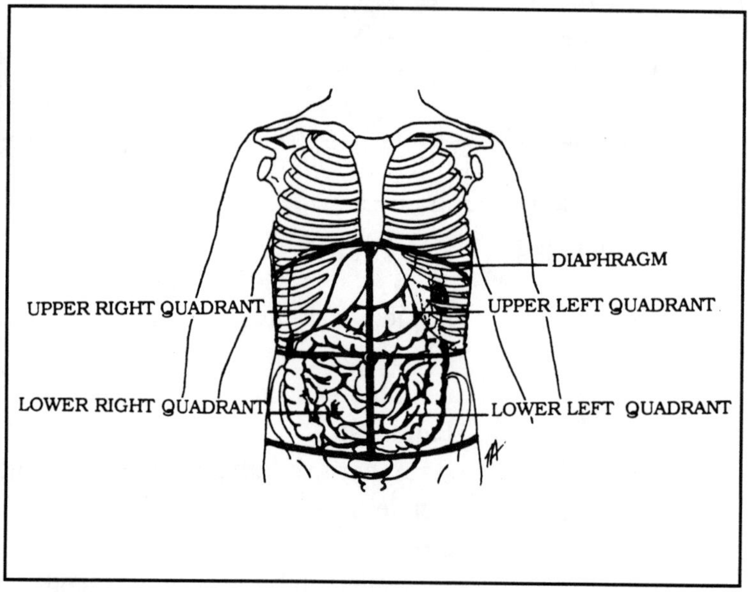

figure 6-10. Abdominal quadrant locations and the organs therein. Use the intersection at the "belly button" as a reference when determining quadrant boundries.

WIND KNOCKED OUT

MECHANISM OF INJURY:

Spasm of diaphragm resulting from an impact to the abdominal area.

PREVENTIVE TREATMENT:

Although athletes are susceptible to having the wind knocked out of them, you can lessen the possibility of injury by not permitting players to have things such as gum, sunflower seeds, tobacco, etc. in their mouths. These items can contribute to choking if they are inhaled when the wind is knocked out of them.

TECHNIQUE FOR TREATMENT:

1. Calm the athlete.
2. While calming and reassuring the athlete, encourage him or her to take small shallow breaths.
3. Loosen any tight clothing. Be careful about lifting up a belt, however, because of possible internal injury to the kidney or spleen.
4. Remove the victim from the event until he or she recuperates fully and there are no signs of internal injuries.

6.7 INJURIES TO EXTREMITIES

Extremities are the most vulnerable parts of the body for injury. Because of the great number of injuries in these areas, it is extremely important to be able to recognize these common injuries.

SHOULDER INJURIES

Shoulder Separation

MECHANISM OF INJURY:

The humerus, or upper arm bone, is forced up through the top of the shoulder, separating the clavicle from the scapula, or a direct blow on the top of the shoulder separates the clavicle from the scapula, causing a shoulder sprain.

figure 6-11. Direction of forces that can cause shoulder separation.

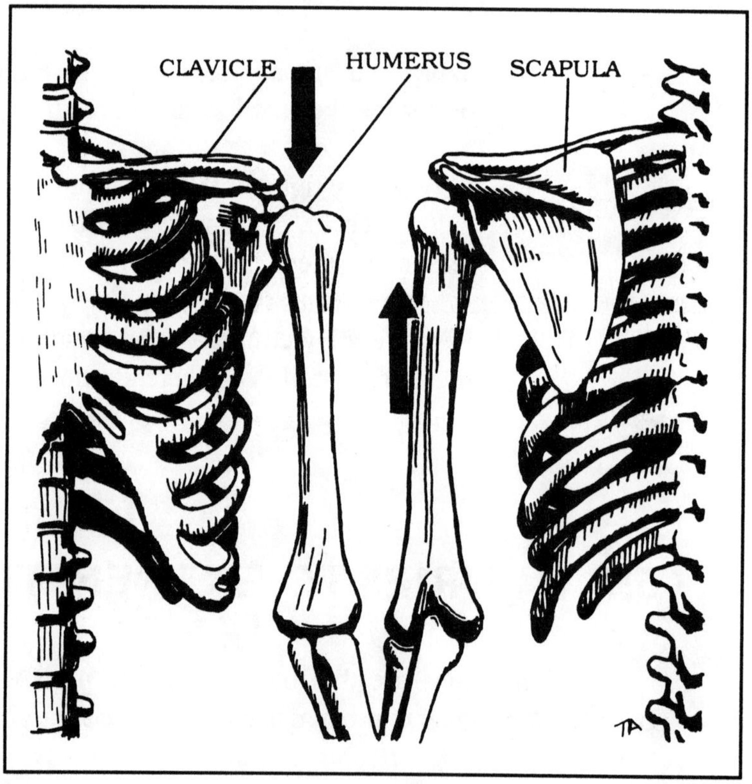

SIGNS/SYMPTOMS:

•Pain and separation at A-C (acromioclavicular) joint when humerus is pushed up through shoulder

•Swelling on top of the shoulder
•Clavicle is protruding upward
•Difficulty moving arm.

TECHNIQUE FOR TREATMENT:

1. Apply R-I-C-E treatment immediately (p. 164).

2. Support arm by placing elbow and arm in a sling (p. 110).

3. Take victim to the emergency room.

Shoulder Dislocation

MECHANISM OF INJURY:

Arm is forced past its normal range of motion and the tip of the humerus is forced out of joint.

SIGNS/SYMPTOMS:

•Deformity of shoulder joint
•Athlete lets arm dangle down at side to avoid pain
•Flattened side of shoulder joint
•Head of humerus can be felt out of joint.

TECHNIQUE FOR TREATMENT (for dislocations):

1. Apply ice to injury. (p. 164)

2. *Do not attempt to reduce dislocation.* This should only be done by a physician.

3. Splint the body part in the same position you found it. Try to make the athlete as comfortable as possible.

*Treatment continued on next page.

4. *TRANSPORT THE VICTIM TO THE EMERGENCY ROOM IMMEDIATELY. TIME IS CRITICAL.* Keep in mind that the physician will need a medical release form to treat the athlete.

Shoulder Rotator Cuff Injury

MECHANISM OF INJURY:

An injury to one or more of the four rotator cuff muscles that hold the humerus in the joint socket and rotate the arm. Caused by violent pulling, swinging or throwing motion of the arm.

SIGNS/SYMPTOMS:

•Pain
•Sharp pain associated with movement, primarily raising the arm overhead or to the side and during throwing follow-through.

Apply **Rotator Cuff Drop Arm Test**: Have athlete place arms straight out to the side and place your hand on the top of the arm. Apply downward resistance. Decreased resistance on the injured side indicates rotator cuff strain.

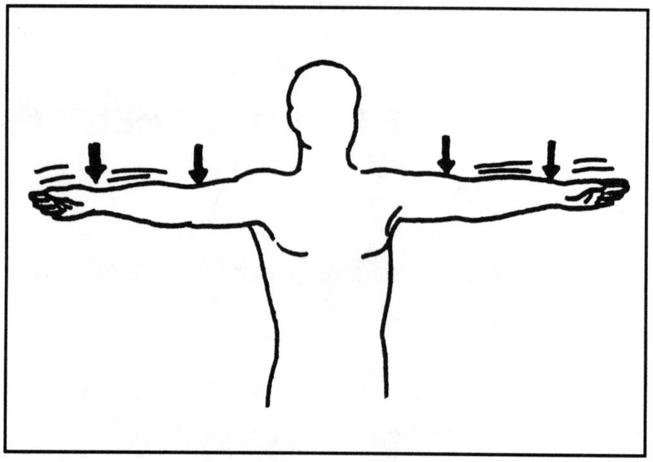

figure 6-12. Positioning of arms for rotator cuff drop arm test.

TECHNIQUE FOR TREATMENT:

1. Apply R-I-C-E treatment (p. 164).
2. Refer to muscular-tendinous treatments (p. 120).

ELBOW INJURIES

Elbow Dislocation

figure 6-13. Bony anatomy of the elbow and forearm.

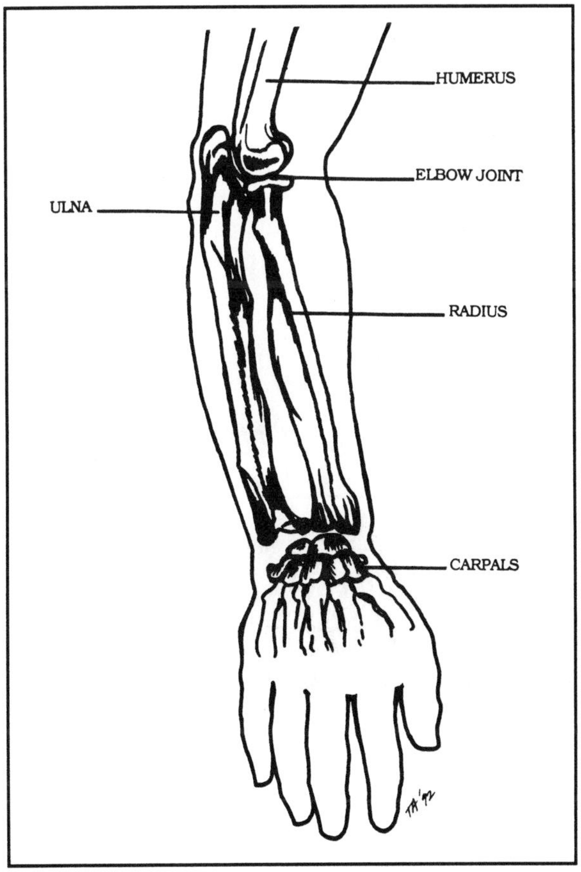

MECHANISM OF INJURY:

Elbow forced out of joint either laterally or medially.

SIGNS/SYMPTOMS:

- •Loss of joint function
- •Deformity
- •Pain.

TECHNIQUE FOR TREATMENT:

Treat as dislocation (p. 151).

Elbow Hyperextension

MECHANISM OF INJURY:

The elbow is forced beyond its normal extension. Usually occurs when an athlete falls upon an outstretched hand with elbow fully extended.

SIGNS/SYMPTOMS:

- Pain in elbow
- A snap or pop
- Painful movement.

TECHNIQUE FOR TREATMENT:

1. Apply R-I-C-E treatment (p. 164).
2. *Always suspect a fracture.*
3. Sling to prevent excess movement (p. 110).
4. Refer to a physician.

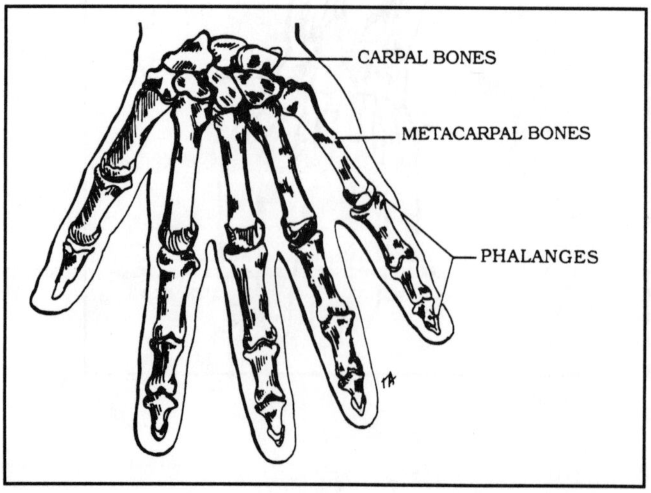

figure 6-14. Bony anatomy of the hand and fingers.

HAND AND FINGER INJURIES

Finger Dislocation

MECHANISM OF INJURY:

Finger hyperextended and forced out of joint by violent force.

SIGNS/SYMPTOMS:

•Loss of function
•Pain or swelling
•Deformity.

TECHNIQUE FOR TREATMENT:

Treat as dislocation (p.151).

Sprained Thumb, Fingers

MECHANISM OF INJURY:

Overextension of thumbs or fingers usually occurs when athletes slide on the turf or floor and thumb or fingers do not move with the body.

SIGNS/SYMPTOMS:

•Swelling
•Pain, especially pain associated with movement
•Skin discoloration.

TECHNIQUE FOR TREATMENT:

Treat as a sprain (p. 117).

KNEE INJURIES

Collateral Ligament Sprain

figure 6-15. Major structures of the knee. Patella (knee cap) has been removed to expose internal tissues.

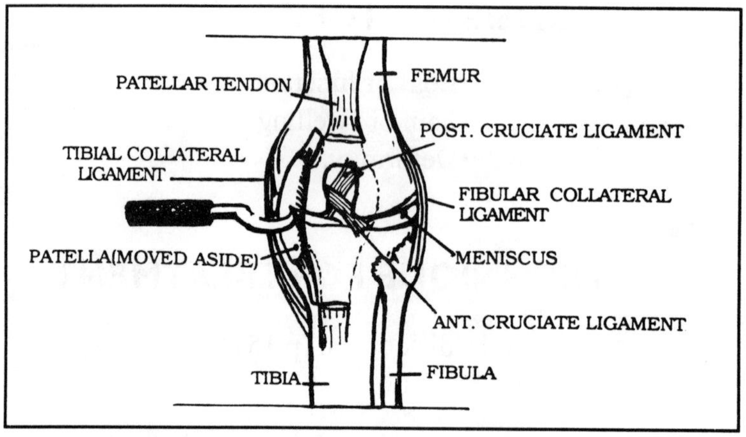

MECHANISM OF INJURY:

A blow to the medial or lateral side of the knee that forces a strain on the collateral ligaments.

SIGNS/SYMPTOMS:

•Medial or lateral looseness
•Swelling
•Pain.

TECHNIQUE FOR TREATMENT:

Treat as a sprain (p. 117).

Twisted Knee

MECHANISM OF INJURY:

Damage to the knee ligaments and/or cartilage. Usually occurs when a foot is planted in the turf and does not rotate when the body twists.

SIGNS/SYMPTOMS:

- Pain
- Swelling
- Partial loss of function
- Inability to bear full weight
- A click or pop in the knee.

TECHNIQUE FOR TREATMENT:

1. Treat as a sprain (p. 117).

2. If the athlete feels extreme pain, treat this injury as a fracture (p. 107).

3. If symptoms persist or if a second or third degree sprain is suspected, take the victim to a physician.

Osgood-Schlatter Disease

CONDITION:

The bony attachment of the patellar tendon is injured and begins recalcification (adding bony tissue). Observed in young athletes.

SIGNS/SYMPTOMS:

figure 6-16. Origin of Osgood-Schlatter pain.

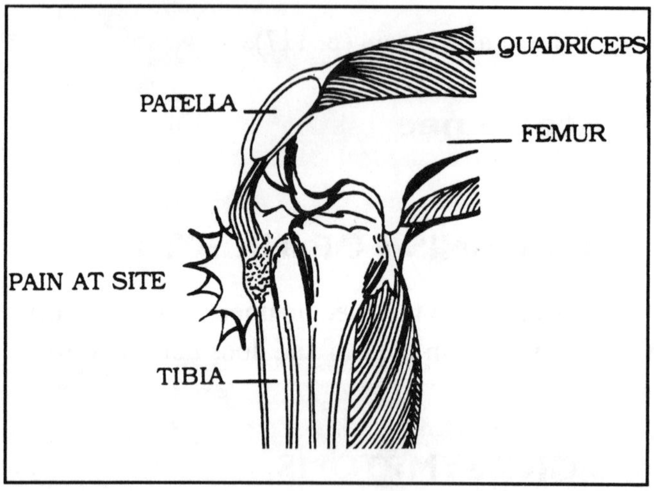

- Swelling
- Pain or tenderness
- Rock-hard swelling just below kneecap (the patellar tendon area)
- Radiating heat from swollen area.

TECHNIQUE FOR TREATMENT:

1. Consult an orthopedic surgeon.
2. Use ice therapy over swollen area (p. 164).
3. Follow medical advice regarding the amount of activity.

LEG, ANKLE AND FOOT INJURIES

Achilles Tendon Strain

MECHANISM OF INJURY:

The foot is forced up (dorsiflexion), which causes a strain on the Achilles tendon.

SIGNS/SYMPTOMS:

figure 6-17. Achilles is injured when foot is forced upwards.

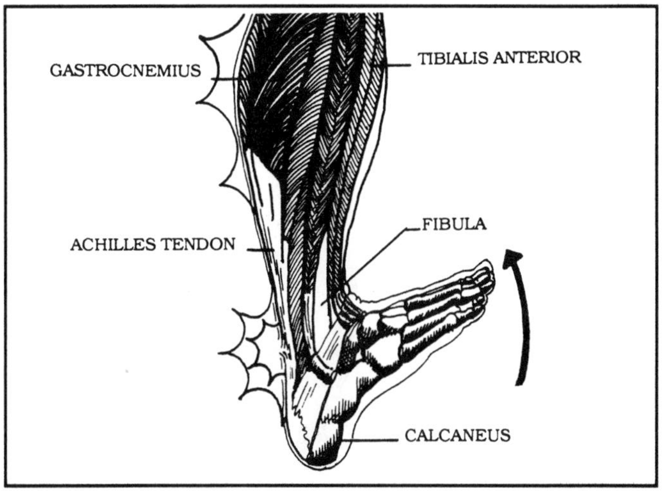

- Soreness on calf (gastrocnemius)
- Swelling
- Pain upon movement.

Apply **Thompson Test**: Place thumb and index finger around the gastrocnemius muscle and squeeze. Plantarflexion of ankle means the Achilles is intact.

TECHNIQUE FOR TREATMENT:

Treat as a strain (p. 120).

Shin Splints

MECHANISM OF INJURY:

Shin splints are usually caused by inflammation of the tibialis posterior muscle, irritation of the bone covering on the tibia in the area associated with the anterior compartment (see figure next page), or irritation of any of the other muscles associated with dorsiflexion and toe extension, such as the tibialis anterior, etc. Poor arch support, muscle imbalance, excessive weight, lack of proper conditioning and stretching, poor running techniques and training "too much, too fast" all can contribute to shin splints.

SIGNS/SYMPTOMS:

•Pain in shin area
•Swelling
•Tenderness.

figure 6-18. Shin splint pain can originate in the tibialis posterior, tibialis anterior, anterior compartment or the tibia (stress fracture).

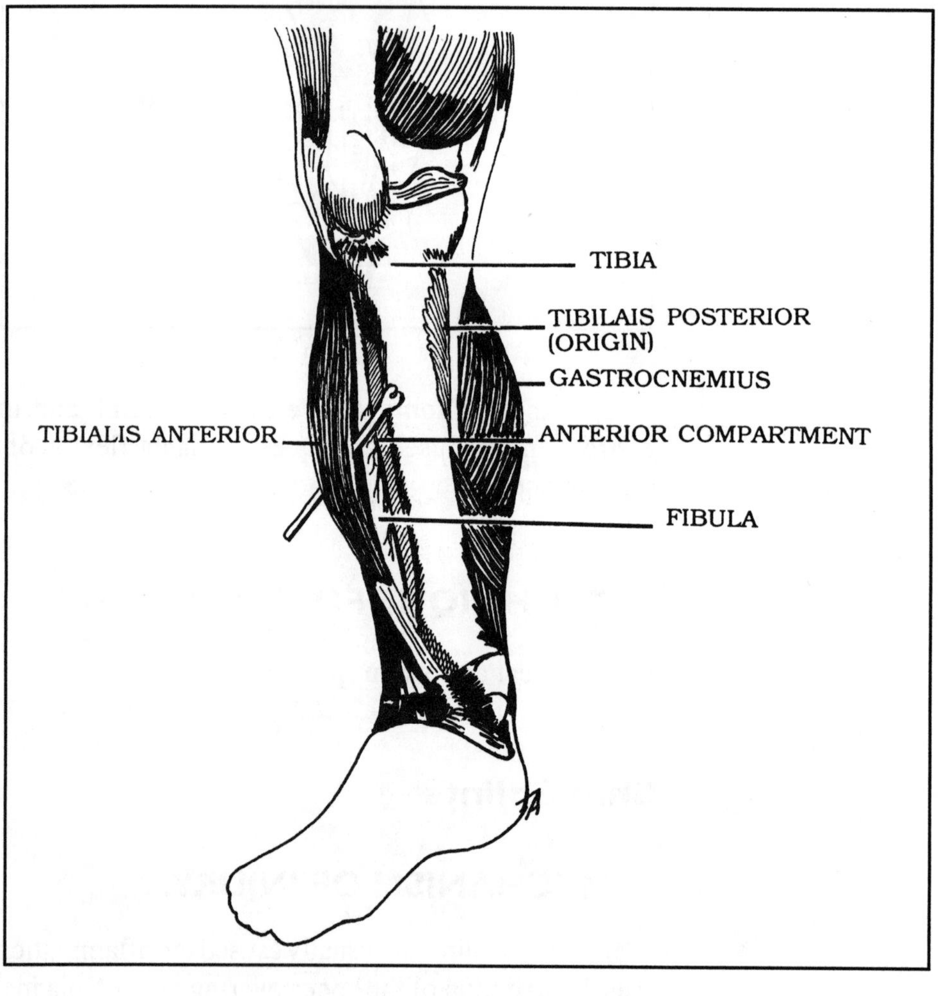

TECHNIQUE FOR TREATMENT:

1. Athletes should be checked for a possible stress fracture if point tenderness is present or if there is chronic pain in one area of the shin.

2. Use ice massage (massage area with ice cubes or a paper cup filled with ice) for 10 minutes. Stretch the shin lightly as often as possible.

3. Continue using ice massage during rest period.

4. Before the next competition, thoroughly warm up the shin area both with heat treatments (p. 165) and activity. If you wish, apply analgesic balm to the area (p. 168) to help decrease discomfort. Stretch and warm up for *at least* 15 minutes. Flexible bandage wrap may be used for support during competition.

5. Reapply ice after competition.

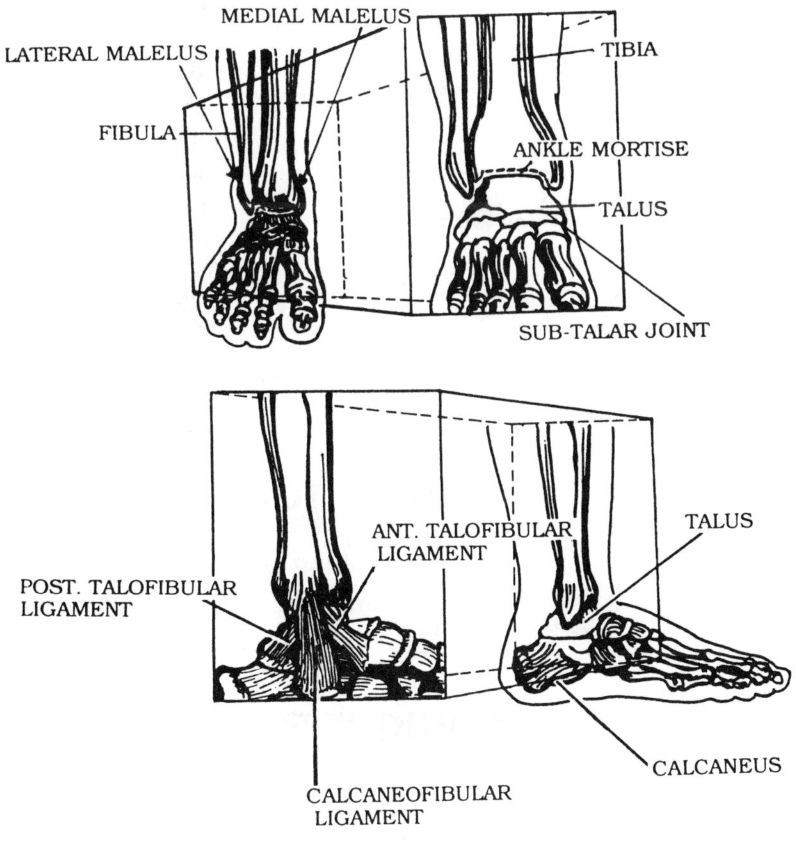

figure 6-19. Ankle anatomy. The anterior talofibular ligament is often sprained in athletic competition.

Sprained Ankle

MECHANISM OF INJURY:

A twist or forced lateral or medial movement exceeding the normal range of motion of the ankle ligaments.

SIGNS/SYMPTOMS:

•Swelling
•Pain
•Skin discoloration (usually reddish/bluish tinge)
•Pain upon movement.

TECHNIQUE FOR TREATMENT:

Treat as a sprain (p. 117).

** *Major sprains are often associated with a fracture.* **

Sprained Toes

MECHANISM OF INJURY:

Overextension of toes. Usually occurs when playing on artificial turf or hard ground with cleats.

SIGNS/SYMPTOMS:

•Swelling
•Pain, pain associated with movement
•Skin discoloration.

TECHNIQUE FOR TREATMENT:

Treat as a sprain (p. 117).

7 Treatments for Minor Sports Injuries

After you have evaluated an injury, it is time to reduce the trauma to the area. Appropriate treatment programs can supplement the body's natural healing powers to restrengthen tissues to their original capacity.

Remember, though, that athletes should not be allowed to participate in sports until they have regained their full strength and support. All coaches and athletes owe it to themselves to have all moderate and serious injuries checked by a trained professional to protect themselves from further injury and liability.

Even though significant advances have been made in sports rehabilitation, the old techniques of cold, heat and stretching are still clearly the best for amateur coaches and athletes. We also cover the use of preparations and taping in this chapter.

7.1 COLD THERAPY (CRYOTHERAPY)

Probably the most valuable tool in the treatment of sports injuries is cold. We will discuss just a few of the many beneficial effects of cold therapy.

Vasoconstriction is probably the most useful attribute of cryotherapy. When a tissue is damaged, the body immediately sends fluids to the damaged tissues. This excessive amount of blood and tissue fluid that accumulates, resulting in the swelling of the tissue, is called **edema**. Ice constricts the blood vessels (vasoconstriction) and capillaries in the tissues and slows the metabolic rate of the muscle, thereby decreasing the fluid flow and retarding edema. Once the edema is controlled, the body can resume natural healing.

The cold temperatures of ice or cold spray penetrate deep into the tissues. Extreme cold desensitizes the nerve endings to reduce irritation and pain. In addition to reducing nerve sensitivity, ice also has been used to decrease muscle spasms at the injury site.

When using ice in first aid, the most effective method of application is the R-I-C-E technique.

R-I-C-E TREATMENT

R=rest	Have athlete rest.
I = ice	Place cold packs or crushed **ice** in a bag on the injury site to reduce swelling and pain.
C = compression	Wrap a moist flexible bandage wrap snugly around the ice and injury to provide **compression**. The athlete should feel some pressure, which constricts the flow of fluids to the injured area.
E = elevation	If no fractures or serious injuries are suspected, **elevate** the injury above heart level. Elevation reduces blood pressure at the injury site.

You'll want to take some precautionary measures with this treatment, however:

1. Do not elevate or move a body part without proper splinting if you suspect a fracture or serious injury.

2. Even if there is no pain in the affected structure, the injury may be serious and should be treated as such.

TECHNIQUE FOR TREATMENT:

1. Apply ice to the injury site as soon as possible, and continue for 48 hours after the trauma.

2. Place at least one layer of protection between the ice and the skin.

3. The athlete receiving the treatment should be as relaxed and comfortable as possible.

4. The injured area should be elevated slightly above the heart when possible.

*Treatment continued on next page.

5. Apply R-I-C-E for 20 minutes. After 20 minutes, remove the ice, but keep the flexible bandage wrap on and continue to elevate the injury. You may reapply the ice after a 20-minute break, (i.e., 20 minutes on, 20 minutes off). Be sure to remove the flexible bandage wrap before bedtime.

6. If there is any question of a fracture, or serious ligament, tendon or muscle damage, continue R-I-C-E treatment, and transport the athlete immediately to the hospital.

7. If swelling or point tenderness persists longer than 72 hours, refer the athlete to a physician.

8. You may apply ice as a chemical cold pack, ice pack, ice massage, etc. Chemical cold packs, however, do not seem to be as effective as ice packs.

7.2 HEAT THERAPY (THERMOTHERAPY)

Current research shows that heat significantly raises the body's resting metabolic rate. When a muscle's metabolic rate increases, its need for oxygen also rises, so the body rushes more blood to the muscle to try to keep up with its increased oxygen demand. With the increased blood flow also comes nutrients, which are needed for tissue repair. That's why heat is so valuable for **vasodilation**, which enhances the rehabilitation of muscle injuries.

Heat should *not* be used, however, until the swelling from the initial trauma has subsided. This could be 48 to 72 hours after the injury occurred. If the swelling has not diminished in 72 hours, consult a physician.

You can apply heat in many forms, including moist heat packs, heating pads, hot baths and whirlpools. You can purchase moist heat packs made from processed silica gel that holds water and steam for about 20 minutes. Moist heat is more effective than dry heat because it penetrates farther.

TECHNIQUE FOR TREATMENT:

1. When using heat, choose a comfortable position so the athlete can remain relaxed for the length of the treatment. The heat packs should rest on top of body parts, so for shoulders, for example, the athlete should sit in a chair with arms supported; for the back, the athlete should be lying prone with a pillow under the abdomen. *If the athlete is lying down and using heat treatments, always elevate the legs. When treatment is complete, the athlete should stand up very slowly.*

2. Always place *at least* one layer of toweling between the heat pack and the athlete. Athletes who have more sensitive skin, such as those with fair complexions, may require more layers.

3. Avoid having the athlete lie on the heat pack. This produces unnecessary wear on the pack, and can constrict blood flow to certain parts of the body.

4. Treat for approximately 20 minutes.

5. Constantly monitor the athlete during treatment.

6. If no progress is made within 72 hours, consult a physician or physical therapist.

WHIRLPOOL TREATMENT:

1. Heat the whirlpool to approximately 106 degrees.

2. Athlete should enter the whirlpool slowly, making sure the injured part is fully immersed.

3. Try not to immerse unnecessary body parts in the whirlpool.

4. Adjust the jet so that it does not propel water directly at the injury site, but hits it at a 45 degree angle.

5. The maximum treatment time should be 20 minutes.

*Treatment continued on next page.

6. Monitor the athlete constantly during treatment.

7. After treatment is completed, the athlete should stand up slowly because blood pools in the immersed parts and cuts down the circulation to the rest of the body.

8. If no progress is made within 72 hours, consult a physician or physical therapist.

7.3 STRETCHING

DEVELOPING A FULL RANGE OF MOTION

The first step in treating an injury is relieving any associated physical and mental trauma. This is often accomplished by simply controlling the swelling and reassuring the athlete. Once the injury has been properly evaluated and determined to not be serious, the second step is to regain the original range of motion of the muscle or joint. As you probably recall, the amount of movement or the number of degrees the body part is able to move from a straight position is called the range of motion, or ROM.

The normal range of motion can be observed by testing the corresponding uninjured body part (providing, of course, that the corresponding uninjured part has not been injured or disabled in the past. If so, corrective surgery or permanent destruction from serious injuries can prohibit full function and make this test invalid.) Regardless, do not bend a joint or muscle past its anatomical limit or past a point that is painful to the athlete.

If the full range of motion is not regained quickly, permanent scar tissue will develop and the athlete will need professional therapy. ROM should be regained by continually moving the joint in increasing ranges of movement by an athlete's *own* strength, not external forces from coaches or parents. If external force is needed or if there is any question about the normal mechanics or extent of the injury, consult a physician immediately.

7.4 ISOMETRICS AND LIGHT EXERCISE

Even if an athlete is immobilized because of an injury, it is important that the rest of that person's body does not weaken and atrophy. Athletes can lose valuable cardiovascular fitness and muscle tone by not staying active.

Take, for example, an athlete with a third degree sprain of his calcaneofibular ligament in his ankle. While his ankle is healing, there are many things he can do to preserve some of his previously attained fitness. First, for proper rehabilitation of the ankle, the surrounding muscles must be kept strong so the ligaments can tighten as quickly as possible. **Isometric exercises** are valuable tools for building static strength. They cause the muscle fibers to contract without shortening, which produces a strain on muscles without moving the body part. Isometrics are usually accomplished by applying a resistive force to prevent the body part from moving during contraction. This prevents further damage to the injured area and keeps the surrounding muscular and tendinous tissues strong.

It is also important to keep the cardiovascular system in good shape. Light exercise raises the regular resting body metabolism by more than 300%. It is an extremely beneficial way to preserve fitness throughout rehabilitation. Some good examples of exercising with a sprained ankle, for instance, are swimming (if the ankle is well-supported), push-ups, chair dips and even hopping on one foot.

There are many ways athletes can stay in shape while rehabilitating an injury, but it is important to consult a physical therapist, athletic trainer or other Sports Medicine professional before attempting isometrics and other rehabilitation exercises.

7.5 PREPARATIONS

ANALGESIC BALMS

Analgesic balms can be beneficial before practice for prevention and for rehabilitation.

Analgesics provide two desired effects:

- Provides a skin irritant, which increases blood flow to the area.

•Relieves pain associated with muscular aches and cramps.

Do not apply analgesics near an open wound or near swollen muscles.

TECHNIQUE FOR TREATMENT:

1. Use a tongue depressor to apply an adequate amount of analgesic cream or oil to the injured area. Massage the area while working in the analgesics to further relax the muscles.

2. Place a towel or a piece of combine roll over the injured area and secure it in place with elastic wrap or athletic tape. (If the tape or wrap tends to slip, spray an adjacent untreated area with tape adherent.)

Current research questions analgesic balms' ability to irritate an area enough to significantly increase blood flow. Studies have shown that the balms' penetration depth is less than one inch, which has little effect on deep muscle tissues. So, most experts agree that the best way to increase blood flow is to increase the inner core temperature of muscle through warm-up exercises.

ANALGESIC AND ANTI-INFLAMMATORY DRUGS

Analgesic drugs reduce pain temporarily, while anti-inflammatory drugs reduce swelling by inhibiting some part of the inflammation process. Many drugs have both analgesic and anti-inflammatory properties, and therefore are used often in athletic injuries. Nonetheless, coaches should never administer any drug to athletes, and we do not encourage or discourage using anti-inflammatory and analgesic drugs in sports. Because many athletes use these drugs, however, it is important that athletes understand their positive and negative effects. Coaches also can discuss the effects of these drugs, leaving the ultimate decision of treatment to the athletes, their parents and their physicians.

Analgesic Drugs

There are many forms of analgesic drugs, from aspirin to narcotics such as morphine, heroine and codeine. Three classes of analgesics can be purchased without a prescription. The decision of which type is best for the athlete should be left to a physician. However, in light of the fact that many analgesics will be used without consulting a physician, a brief introduction of each drug type is included below.

ACETYLSALICYLATE BASED DRUGS

This class includes aspirin and related drugs that contain salicylates. In the United States alone, more than 55 million pounds of aspirin-related drugs are ingested annually. Every year, there are more than 150,000 serious or fatal cases of aspirin poisoning.

Aspirin is an **analgesic** drug, or "pain killer," that is often used to relieve the pain associated with arthritis, sprains, strains and tendinitis. Aspirin is also an **anti-inflammatory** drug that slows the release of **prostaglandins**, which stimulate inflammation. When prostaglandin release slows, swelling decelerates. Aspirin also acts as an **antipyretic**, reducing fever in the body.

On the negative side, many frequent users of aspirin develop gastrointestinal hemorrhaging. This can lead to ulcers, nausea, intestinal and other digestive problems. Aspirin also increases fluid loss from the body by stimulating the sweating process, which promotes water loss, especially if used daily. Through its effect on the kidneys, it may also stimulate urinary output, which can lead to a deficiency of potassium and sodium, elements that are crucial for proper fluid balance in the body. Aspirin also increases bleeding by delaying clotting and has been shown to trigger asthma attacks for some asthmatics. Finally, aspirin has been shown to depress thirst in athletes. For these reasons, athletes should exercise extra caution in using aspirin during competition, especially during hot weather.

As with any drug, adverse reactions may occur at doses smaller than those recommended by the manufacturer. If any of the following symptoms occur, immediately discontinue use of product and consult a physician.

SIGNS/SYMPTOMS:

- Headache

- •Ringing in ears
- •Dizziness
- •Drowsiness
- •Any unusual or exaggerated allergic reaction (anaphylaxis)
- •Skin irritation (eruption)
- •Asthma
- •Vomiting
- •Sweating.

IBUPROPHEN BASED DRUGS

Ibuprophen basically has the same properties as aspirin. Athletes who have allergic reactions to aspirin *should not* use this product. Some aspirin-sensitive athletes find ibuprophen reduces gastric discomfort.

ACETAMINOPHEN BASED DRUGS

Acetaminophen drugs include products such as Tylenol™ and Aspirin Free Excedrin™. They have analgesic and strong antipyretic properties with very few side effects. Most athletic injuries, however, involve inflammation, and acetaminophen has no anti-inflammatory properties. So, athletes who are sensitive to salicylate and ibuprophen often use these drugs to ease pain. This is usually the drug of choice in fever reduction. Gastric irritation is usually not noted in acetaminophen use.

table 7-1. Properties of various analgesic drugs. Product names listed are registered trademarks of their respective companies.

	SALICYLATES	ACETAMINOPHEN	IBUPROPHEN
PRODUCT NAMES	ANACIN BAYER	TYLENOL, ASPIRIN FREE EXCEDRIN	MOTRIN ADVIL NUPRIN
ANALGESIC	YES	YES	YES
ANTI-INFLAMMATORY	YES	NO	YES
ANTI-PYRETIC	YES	YES	YES

Anti-Inflammatory Drugs

Anti-inflammatory drugs can be divided into two types: steroidal anti-inflammatories (SAI) and non-steroidal anti-inflammatories (NSAI). SAI drugs resemble the glucocortical steroids produced in the adrenal medulla (see the information on the Endocrine System, p. 31). Because of their potential side effects, all SAIs are dispensed by prescription only, except for some topical hydrocortisones. NSAI drugs include aspirin, ibuprophen and a host of other prescription drugs.

table 7-2. Various anti-inflammatory medications. Product names listed are registered trademarks of their respective companies.

NSAIs	SAIs
MOTRIN	ARISTOCORT
NAPROSYN	CORTONE ACETATE
INDOCIN	DECADRON
FELDENE	HYDROCORTONE
NUPRIN	HYDROCORTIZONE
ANSAID	MEDROL
ADVIL	PREDNISONE

The use of DMSO (dimethyl sulfoxide) is not recommended for humans.

7.5 INTRODUCTION TO ATHLETIC TAPING

There will be very few occasions when an athlete will have a particular joint that is strong enough to compete, yet needs to be supported by tape. It is important to note that taping is *not* a substitute for strong tissues which normally support a joint. If a coach is able to tape a minor injury or chronically weak joint, however, it is often a real confidence-builder for everyone concerned.

Before taping, the coach or Sports Medicine professional should test the injury to make sure it is strong enough to handle the high torque and pressure of competition. If it is strong enough, then tape may be applied to give it further support.

*** IF THERE IS ANY DOUBT ABOUT WHETHER THE JOINT IS STRONG ENOUGH, CONSULT A PROFESSIONAL ATHLETIC TRAINER OR PHYSICIAN. ***

The taper, or person who is taping, should know how to tape properly and be aware of any potential problems. Actually, the art of athletic taping takes considerable practice to master. Improper taping procedures can contribute to uneven pressure in applying the tape, which can cause blisters and soreness.

Follow these steps for athletic taping at all times:

- The athlete should be sitting or standing on a flat surface with the appendage in proper position to be taped.

- The taping table or surface should be of sufficient height so the taper does not need to bend over in an uncomfortable position.

- The taper should stand in front of the appendage to be taped. The taper's feet should be flat on the floor in a comfortable position and with weight evenly distributed.

- Prepare the skin area to be taped by:
    - -Shaving hair (optional)
    - -Using tape adhesive
    - -Applying Vaseline™ pads to critical pressure areas
    - -Using pre-wrap or gauze to cover the skin under tape.

- Apply the tape according to the techniques presented on the subsequent pages.

- Always pull tape up on the side that requires support.

- Be aware of the correct angles of application so that the tape lays flat against the skin.

FINGER TAPING

The easiest way to protect sprained finger joints is with a splint. This has certain limitations in sports, however, so a good substitute for the splint is to tape the injured finger to its neighbor for support.

To tape a finger to another finger [figure 7-1 (1-6)], place a gauze pad between the fingers to be taped together (1). Use two pieces of 1" tape about 8" in length to anchor the fingers together. Put the first piece around the finger between the knuckle and the first joint (2) and the second between the two joints of the finger proper (3). If you need greater stabilization, apply a splint strip of tape, starting from the knuckle on the palm side of the finger, running over the tip of the finger, and ending at the knuckle on the back side of the finger (4). Then apply the circular support strips as previously described. This additional strip better restricts the flexion and extension motions in the finger joints (5 and 6).

figure 7-1. Two methods of finger taping.

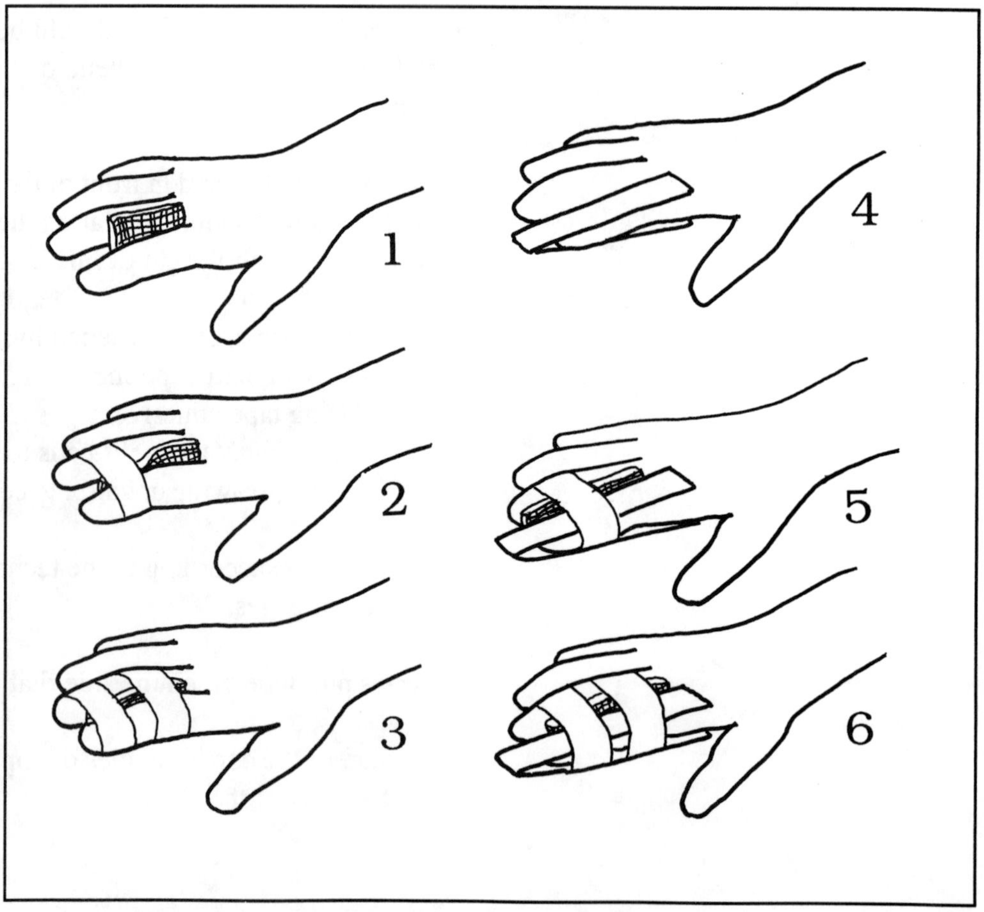

THUMB TAPING

The easiest and safest way to protect a sprained thumb is to tape it to its neighboring finger. However, this poses a problem in many sports because the procedure does not allow grasping. When the athlete does not need an opposable thumb, the butterfly is easiest and most convenient method to protect the thumb. If grasping is required, use the figure-eight method.

Butterfly

With the thumb held approximately 1" from the index finger, wind a strip of 1" tape around the bottom section of the index finger and the end of the thumb [figure 7-2 (1)]. Then wind a small strip of ½" tape around the middle of this tape to pinch it in the center [figure 7-2 (2)] and create the "butterfly" format for which it is named.

Figure-Eight

Figure-eight taping restricts bending away from the hand by wrapping tape around the knuckle of the thumb. You can use pre-taping underwrap around the wrist and the base of the thumb in a figure-eight pattern. The person being taped should hold the hand with the thumb as if about to reach out and pick up a small bottle. Wrap 1" adhesive tape around the wrist and the base of the thumb in the same figure-eight pattern, overlapping most of the strip of the previous turn [figure 7-2 (3-6)]. Be careful to not pull the tape too tight across the fleshy part of the hand between the thumb and first finger. If the thumb darkens in color or begins to feel "funny," loosen or reapply the tape. To increase protection, use a "butterfly" in addition to the "figure-eight."

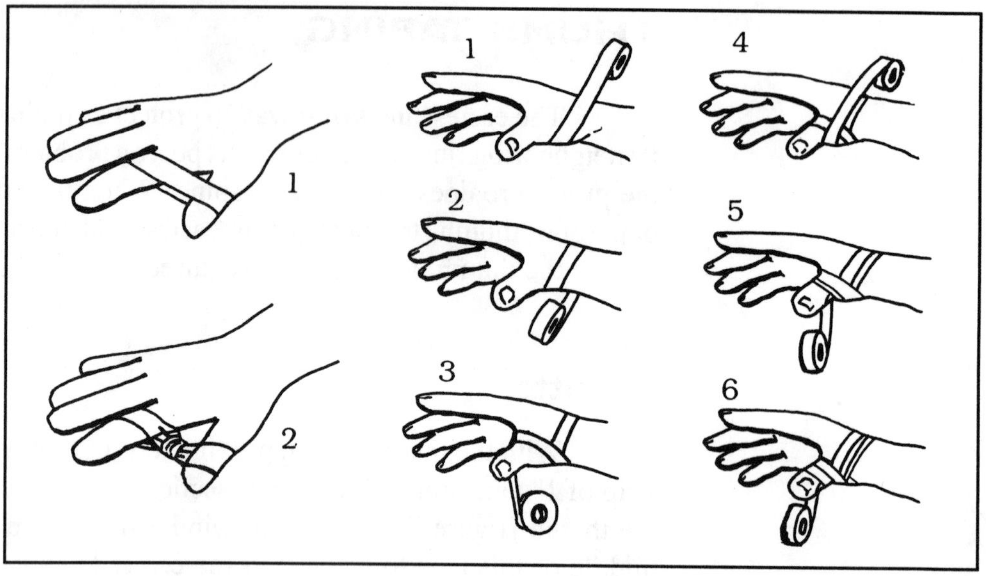

figure 7-2. Thumb taping using the butterfly (left) and figure-8 (right) techniques.

WRIST TAPING

One of the most common and easiest taping procedures is wrapping tape around the wrist. This procedure provides some support and restriction for wrist joint motions. During application, have the person tightly clench the fist of the hand being taped to reduce the possibility of wrapping the tape too tight. First, apply a layer of pre-taping underwrap snugly around the wrist and contour it as far up on the back of the hand as possible without having the edge roll over (figure 7-3). Now apply 1½" adhesive tape, overlapping the previous layer, by circling the wrist five or six complete times.

For more wrist joint support, strip tape across the back of the hand and wrist to protect from bending *down*, across the palm side of the hand and wrist to protect from bending *back*, or both to protect from bending down and back [figure 7-3 (1a-7a)]. Place an anchor strip of 1½" tape around the hand at the knuckle line and a second, 2" to 3" above the wrist bones (closer to the elbow) (1a). Apply parallel and overlapping strips of 1½" tape to the backside and/or palm of the hand from one anchor strip to the other (2a). Five to seven strips will suffice, with the last two applied in an X-pattern to reinforce and better restrict motion (3a through 5a). Now, hold these strips in position by continuous taping around the hand, wrist and lower arm (7a). You can also pre-cut the support strips and position them on a glass or similar smooth surface. Lift these strips as a group, and place them in position between the anchor strips, then tape around as previously described.

figure 7-3. Taping of the wrist and hand.

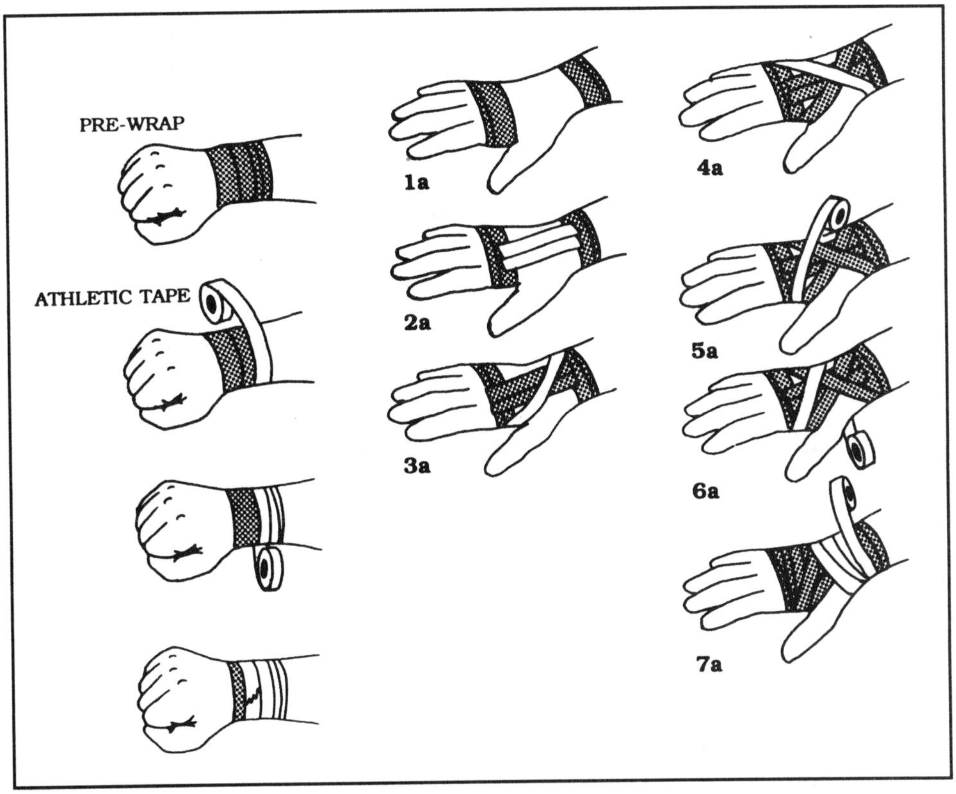

ANKLE TAPING

There are many ways to tape an ankle, but there is a simple procedure that athletes can apply on themselves if they are skillful and flexible enough to reach their own foot and ankle [figure 7-4 (1-23)].

If possible, the athlete should be standing with the ball of the foot to be taped supported on the edge of a chair seat and the ankle at no more than a 90^0 angle. If a coach is doing the taping, the athlete should sit on a table with the ankle dangling over the end in a slightly dorsiflexed position.

Place gauze cushions or 1/8" lubricated felt or foam across the instep and over the Achilles tendon. Hold them in place with pre-taping underwrap (1) by wrapping it from the mid-foot to 4 to 6" above the ankle bones (2). Apply two anchor strips of 1½" tape around the leg at the top edge of the underwrap material (3). Now apply five or six overlapping stirrup strips of 1½" tape from the anchor on the inside of the leg, under the arch, to the anchor on the outside of the leg (4 through 7). Apply the last two of these support strips diagonally, both beginning on the inside of the leg, with one coming forward (8 and 9) and the other going to the rear (10 and 11). Now use a series of locking strips to cover the ends of the support strips and hold them in position, applying them the same way you did the anchor strips, starting at the top and coming down the leg and ending at the ankle bones (12).

Next, apply a heel-locking pattern around the ankle and over the stirrups to increase joint stability. You can do this with standard tape, but elastic tape, pulled snug, is more comfortable and easier to apply. Start this pattern on the outside of the heel (13), carry it over the instep and under the foot and then back to the beginning of the tape. Then wrap it up the heel on the outside (14), around and slightly above the ankle bones (15), down the heel on the inside (16), and then into a figure-eight pattern around the ankle joint (17 and 18). Wrap the tape once more up the heel on the outside (19) and then spiral it up the leg to the top of the stirrup strips (20 through 23). Increase the support by adding additional heel-locking patterns.

Be careful not to bring the tape (stirrups or heel-lock) too far forward on the outer border of the foot. If you put too much pressure over the little bump of bone (the head of the fifth metatarsal), it may begin to ache. Keep the stirrup strips and the circular patterns behind this bony protuberance so you do not create excessive pressure on the outer border of the foot. Overall, the amount of tension will be dictated by comfort, desired amount of support, and the skill of the taper.

figure 7-4. Wrapping and taping of the ankle.

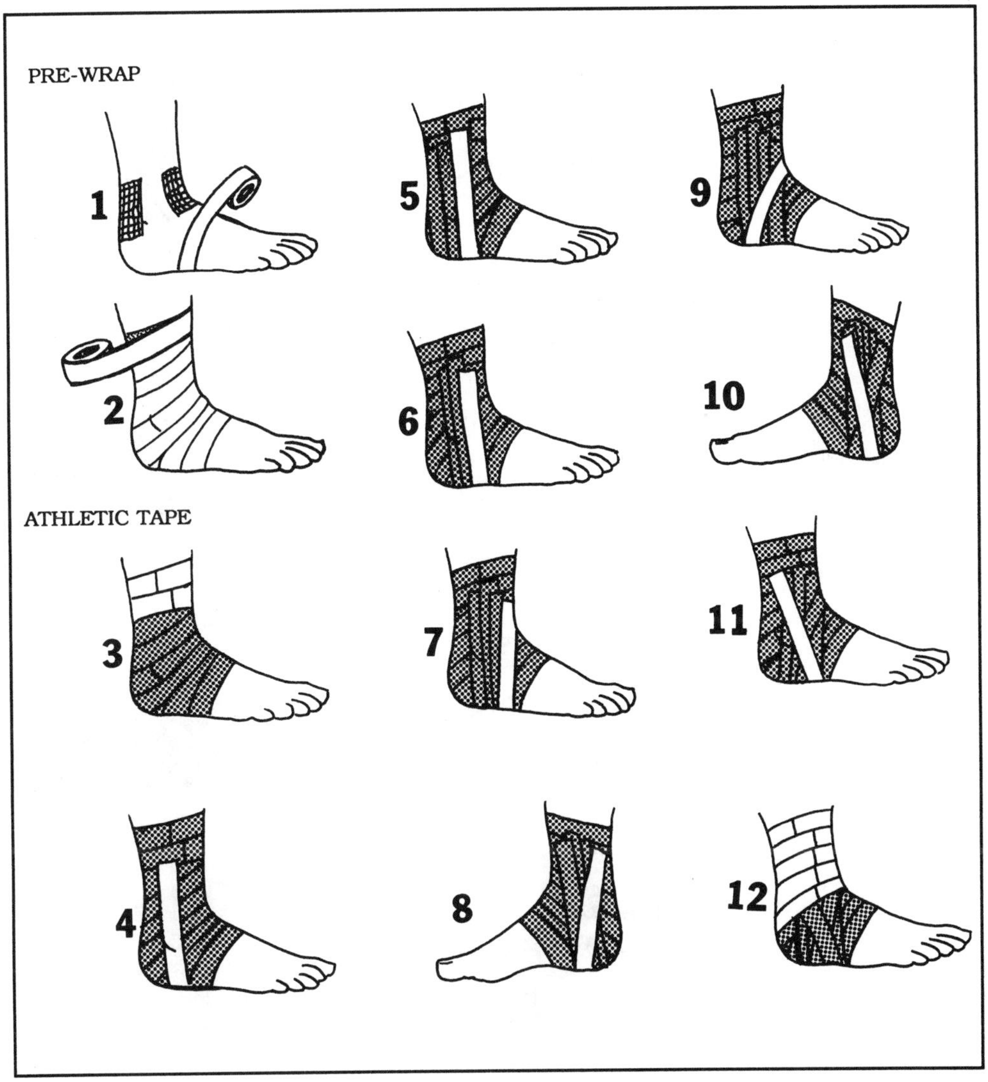

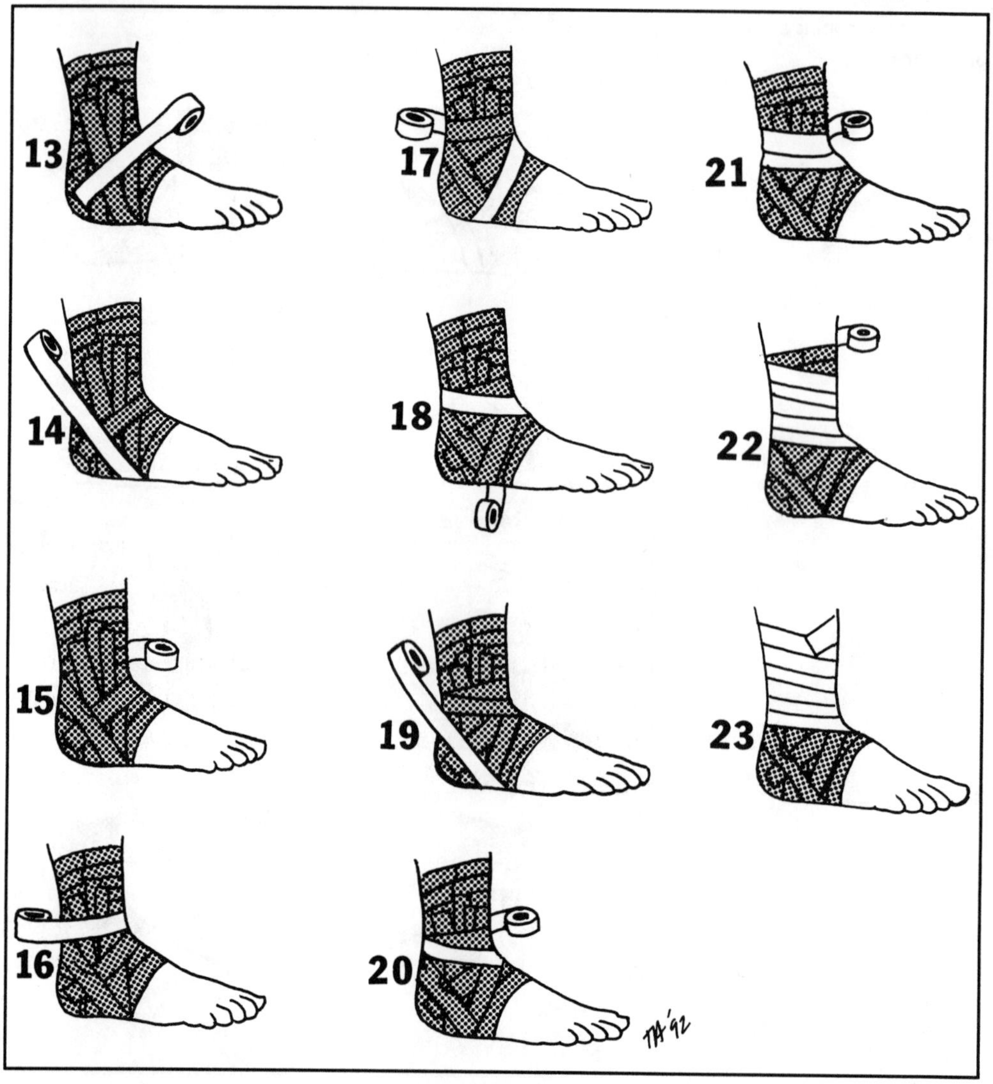

figure 7-4 (cont.). Wrapping and taping of the ankle.

ARCH TAPING

Arch taping can help prevent discomfort in athletes suffering from fallen or weakened arches, shin splints and plantar fascitis. This taping procedure is relatively easy to master [figure 7-5 (1-11)].

To begin, the athlete should be sitting on a table with the foot hanging off the end in a slightly dorsiflexed position. Apply an anchor of 1½" tape so that the top surface is directly above the heads (ends closest to the toe bones) of the first metatarsal (below the big toe) and fifth metatarsal (below the smallest toe) as in (2). Next, apply a heel strip from the anchor strip on the small toe side, around the heel and back to the anchor strip (3).

Now, begin the modified figure-eight patterns by tearing your 1½" tape in half and starting at either the first or fifth toe side. Each strip should parallel the heel strip, pass behind the heel and cross the arch so it ends up at the same place it began (4 and 5). Each *pair* of these strips should form an X across the arch; one modified figure-eight starts at the big toe, while the next starts on the small toe side. These pairs should overlap the previous ones by half (6 and 7). The X patterns should progress from the arch near the heel to near the toes (6 and 7), producing a woven effect.

Next, apply several support strips from the heel strip on the lateral aspect of the foot, across the arch, to the heel strip on the arch side of the foot (8 and 9). Again, overlap each strip halfway on the previous strip. Apply two layers of support strips.

Apply another heel strip (3), followed by another anchor (2), and a couple pieces that cross over the top of the foot to hold the tape in place during movement.

figure 7-5. Taping of the arch.

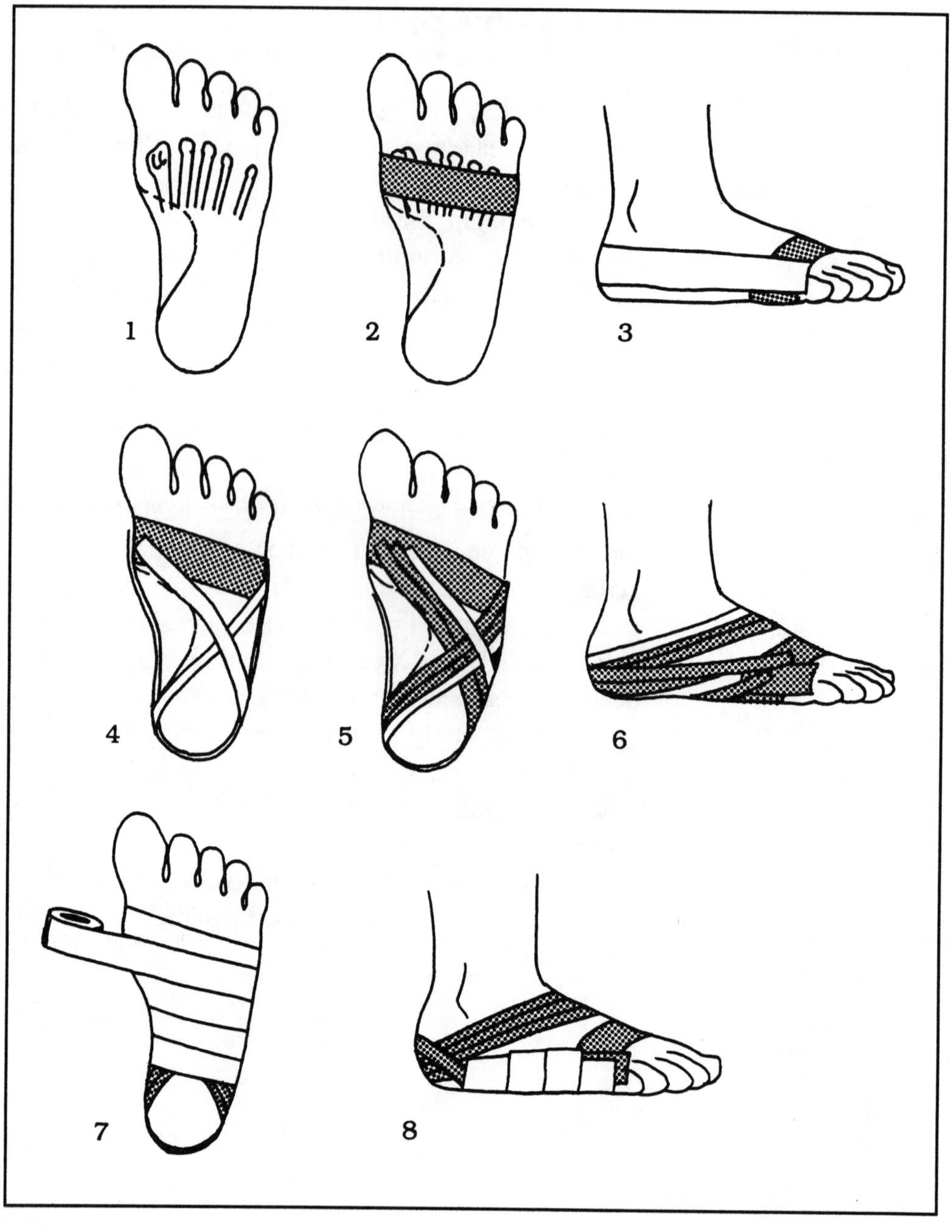

References

1. Abdo, S.C.: "Injury Prevention Through Weight Training—The Balanced Approach," National Strength and Conditioning Association Journal, Jan. 30-31, 1985.

2. Alkinson, J.G., and Andrew, G.M.: The Child in Sport & Physical Activity, Baltimore University Park Press, 1976.

3. American Academy of Pediatrics: "Injuries to Young Athletes," The Physician and Sports Medicine, 9 (2): 107-110, Feb. 1981.

4. American College of Sports Medicine: Guidelines for Exercise Testing and Prescription, Lea and Febriger, Philadelphia, PA, 1986.

5. American Heart Association: The American Heart Association Diet, 7320 Greenville Ave., Dallas, TX, 1985.

6. American Red Cross: Advanced First Aid and Emergency Care: 2nd Ed., 1979.

7. American Red Cross: Multimedia Standard First Aid, 1981.

8. Anderson, B.: Stretching, Shelter Publications, 1980.

9. Bachman, David C.: Dear Dr. Jack, Dutton, 1980.

10. Bailey, C.: The New Fit or Fat, Houghton Mifflin Co., 1991.

11. Fahey, Thomas D.: What to do About Athletic Injuries, Butterick Pub., New York, 1979.

12. Fox, E.L.: Sports Physiology, W.B. Saunders Co., Philadelphia, PA, 1979.

13. Garrick, James: PEAK CONDITION! Winning Strategies to Prevention, Treatment, & Rehabilitation of All Sports Injuries, Crown, New York, 1986.

14. Grant, H.D., Murray, R.H., Bergeron, J.D.: Emergency Care: 3rd Ed., Brady Communications Co. Inc., 1982.

15. Hackworth, C., Jacobs, K., O'Neil, C.: Prevention, Recognition, and Care of Common Sports Injuries, SWM Systems, Inc., 1982.

16. Hossler, P.: Handbook of Athletic Training, Movement Publications, 1983.

17. Johnson & Johnson Products, Inc.: AthletiCare Taping Guide, 501 George St., New Brunswick, NJ, 1985.

18. Kaus, Hans: The Causes, Prevention, and Treatment of Sports Injuries, Playboy Press, New York, 1981.

19. Klafs, Carl E., Arnheim, D.: Modern Principles of Athletic Training, C.V. Mosby Co., St. Louis, MO, 1979.

20. Kravitz, L.: Anybody's Guide To Total Fitness, Kendall/Hunt Publishing Co., Dubuque, IA, 1986.

21. Martens, R., Christina, R.W., Harvey, J.S., and Sharkey, B.J.: "Coaching Young Athletes," Human Kinetics Publishers, Inc., Champaign, IL, 1981.

22. Mirkin, Gabe: The Sports Medicine Book, Little, 1978.

23. O'Donoghue, D.H.: Treatment of Injuries to Athletes, Philadelphia, PA, W.B. Saunders, 1976.

24. Otto, R.M., Fox, E.L., and Stevens, C.J.: "Metabolic Responses of Young Women To Training and Maintenance/Detraining," Medicine and Science in Sports, 10 (1), 52, 1978.

25. Shangold, Mona M.: The Complete Sports Medicine Book For Women, Simon & Schuster, New York, 1985.

26. Smith, N.J.: "Sports Medicine: Health Care for Young Athletes," American Academy of Pediatrics, 1983.

Appendix

COMMON WEIGHT TRAINING EXERCISES

figure A-1. The bench press.

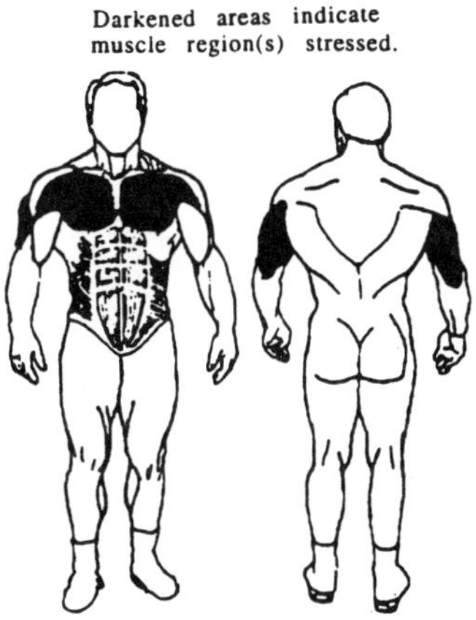

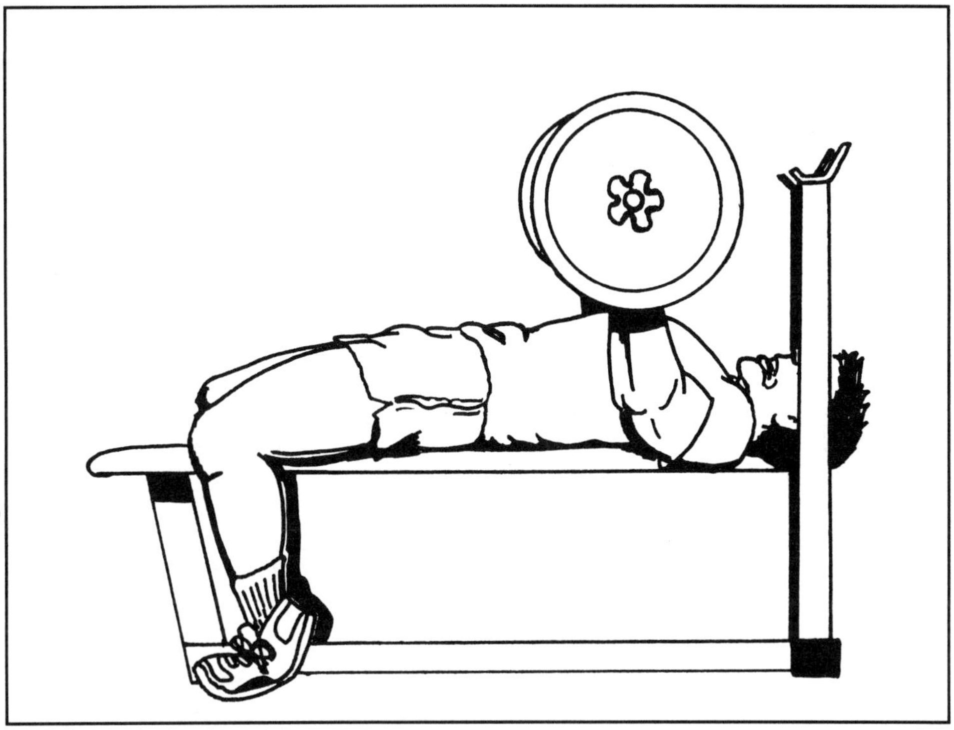

figure A-2. The military press.

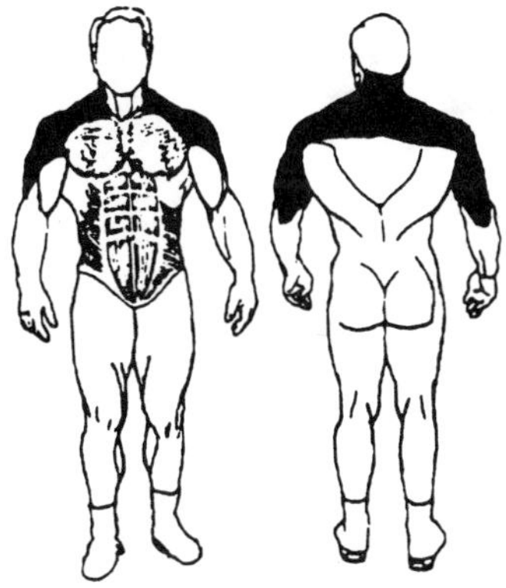

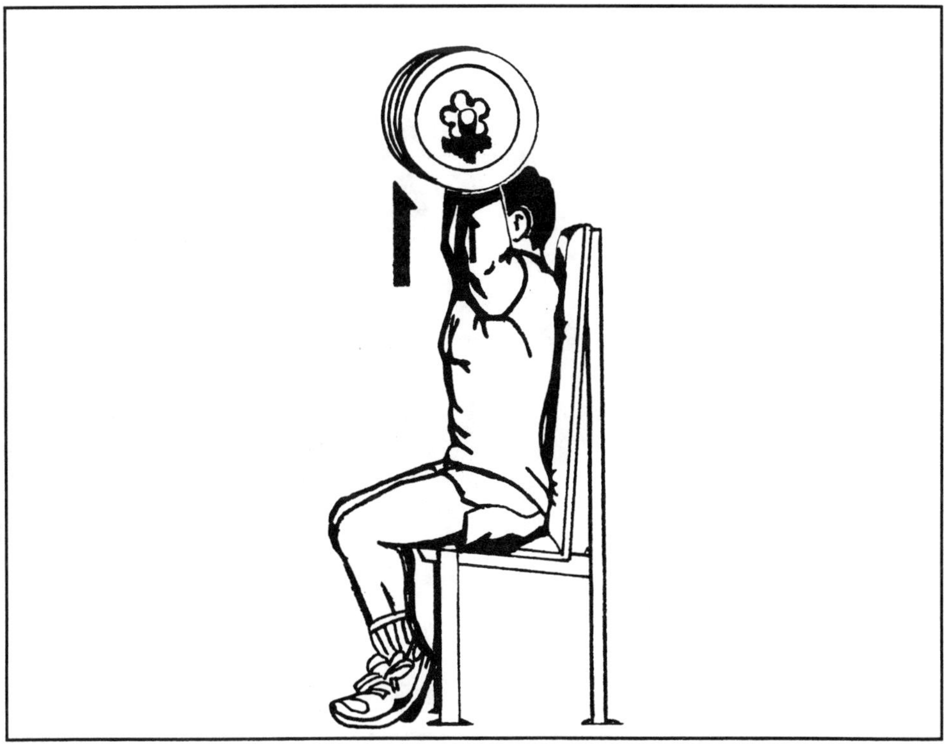

figure A-3. The biceps curl.

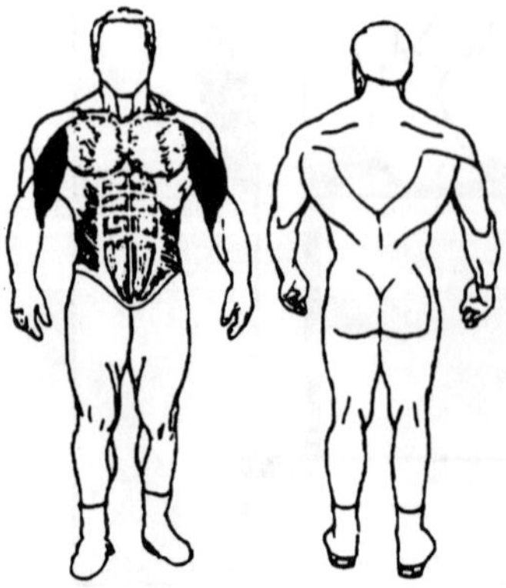

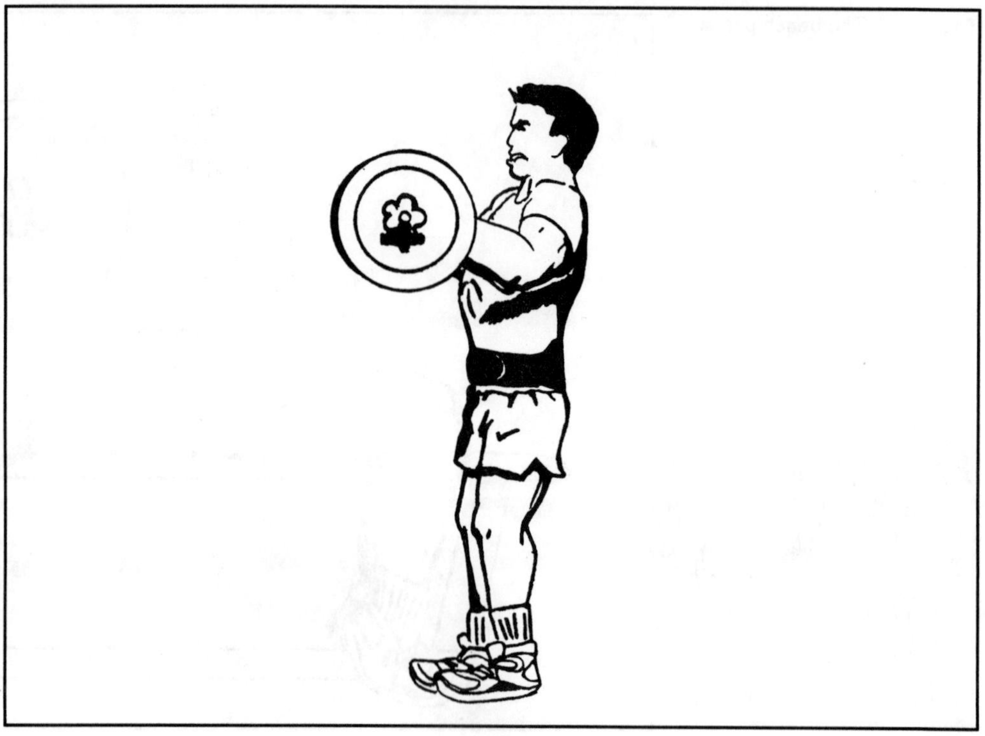

figure A-4. The triceps push-down.

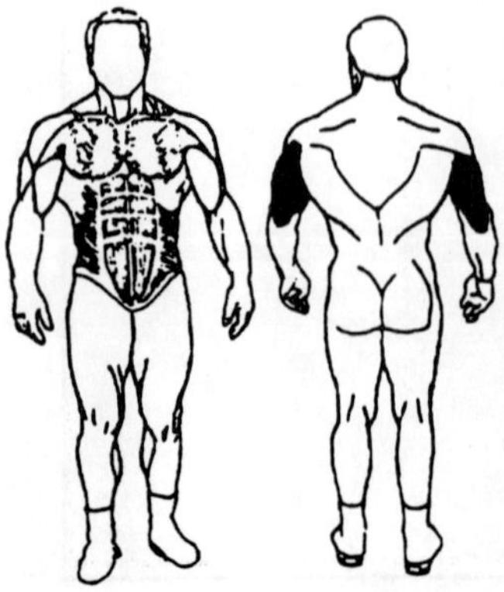

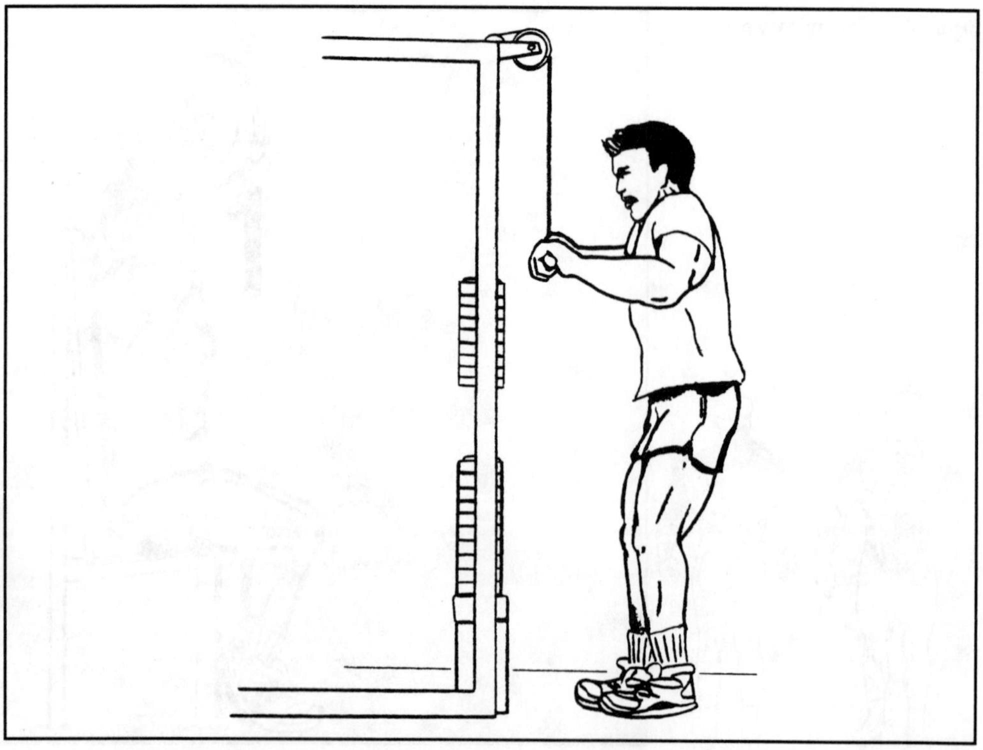

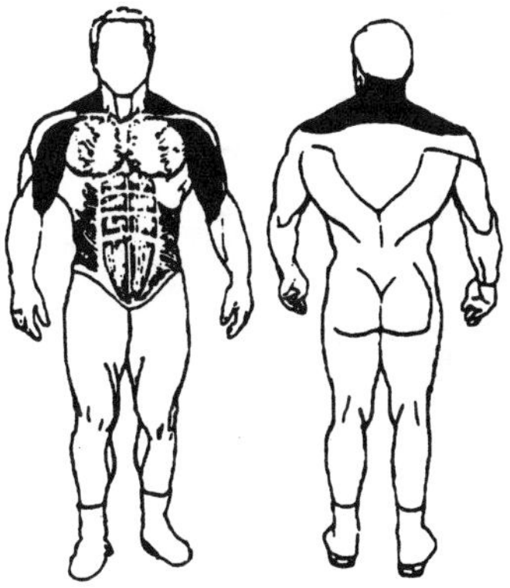

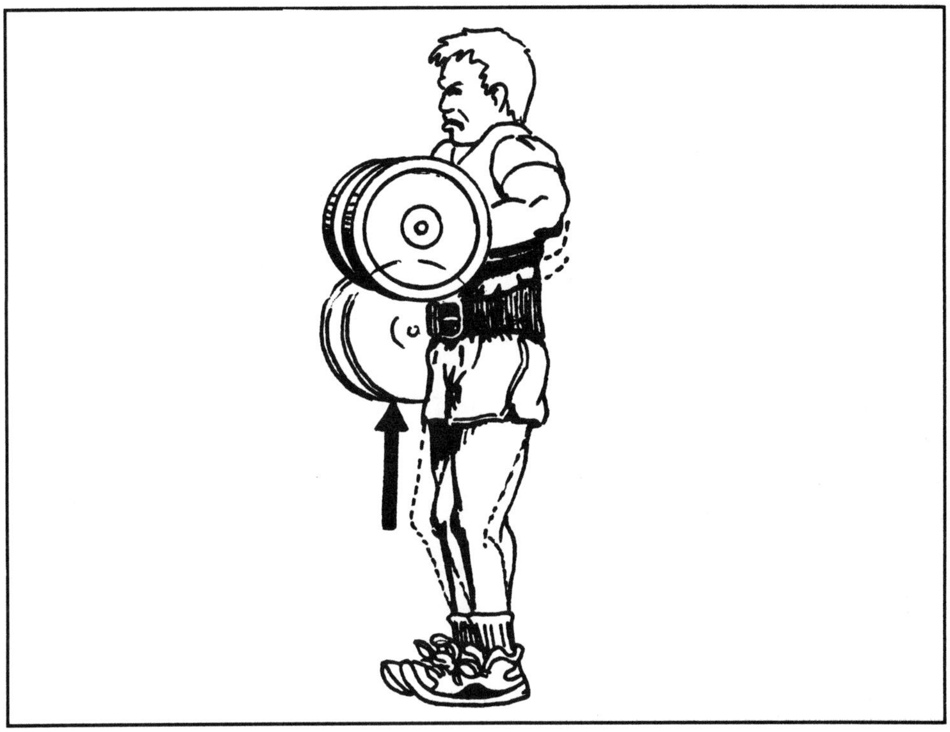

figure A-5. The upright row.

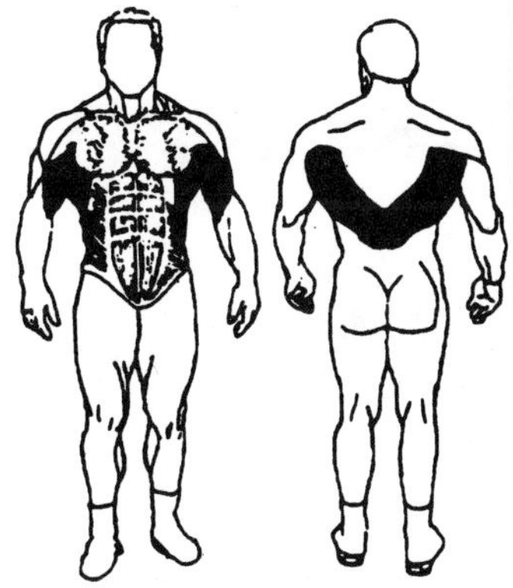

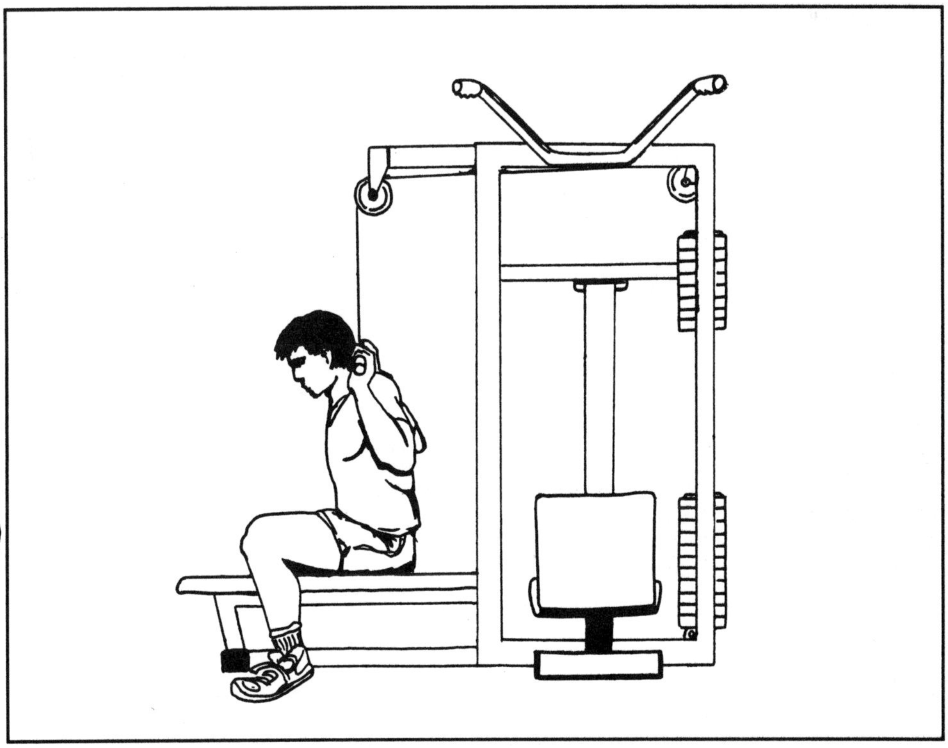

figure A-6. The latissimus dorsi, or "lat", pull-down.

figure A-7. The hamstring, or leg, curl.

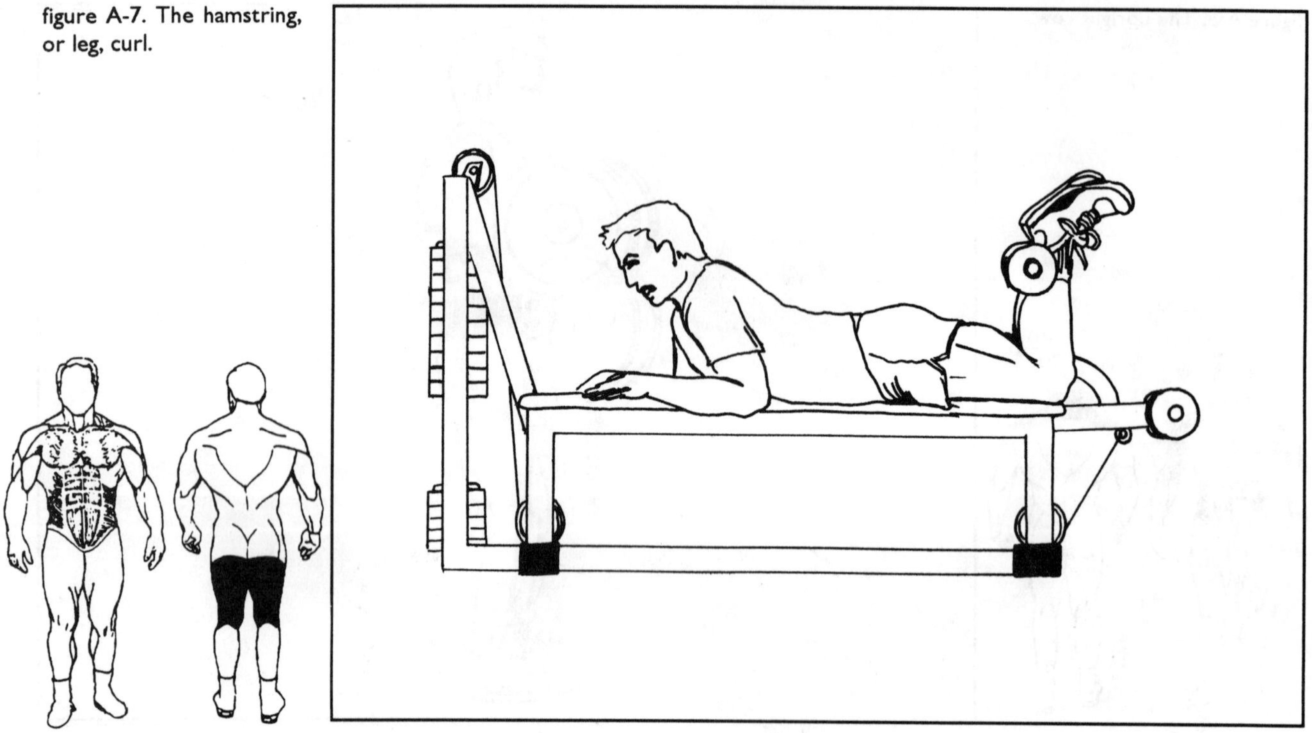

figure A-8. The quadriceps, or leg, extension.

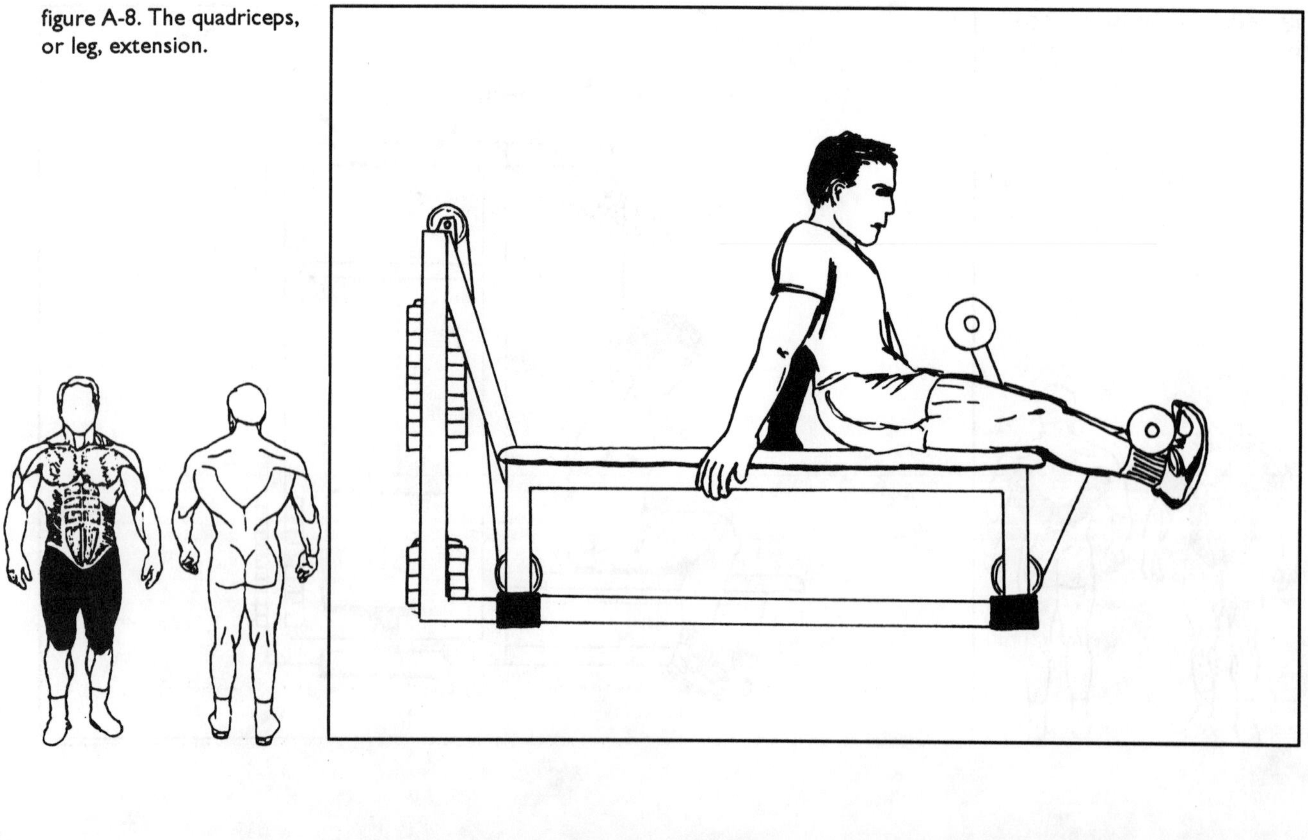

figure A-9. The leg press.

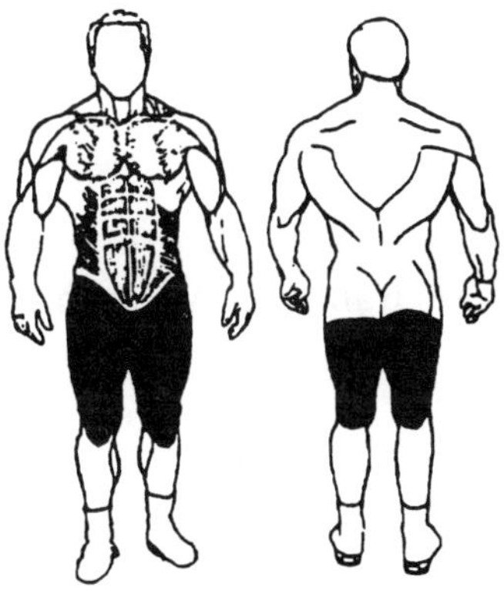
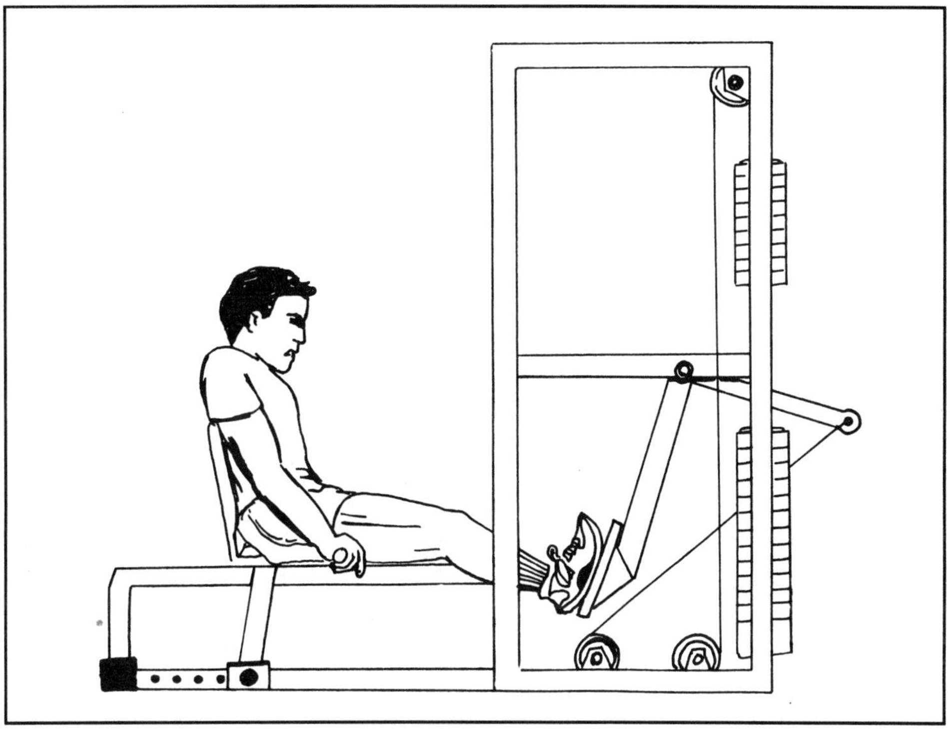

figure A-10. The squat.

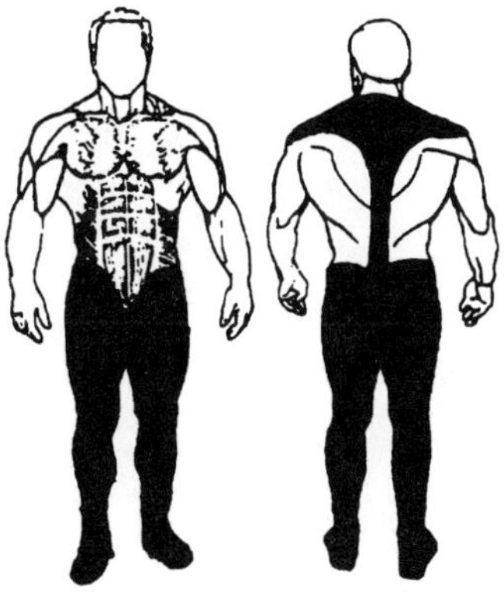
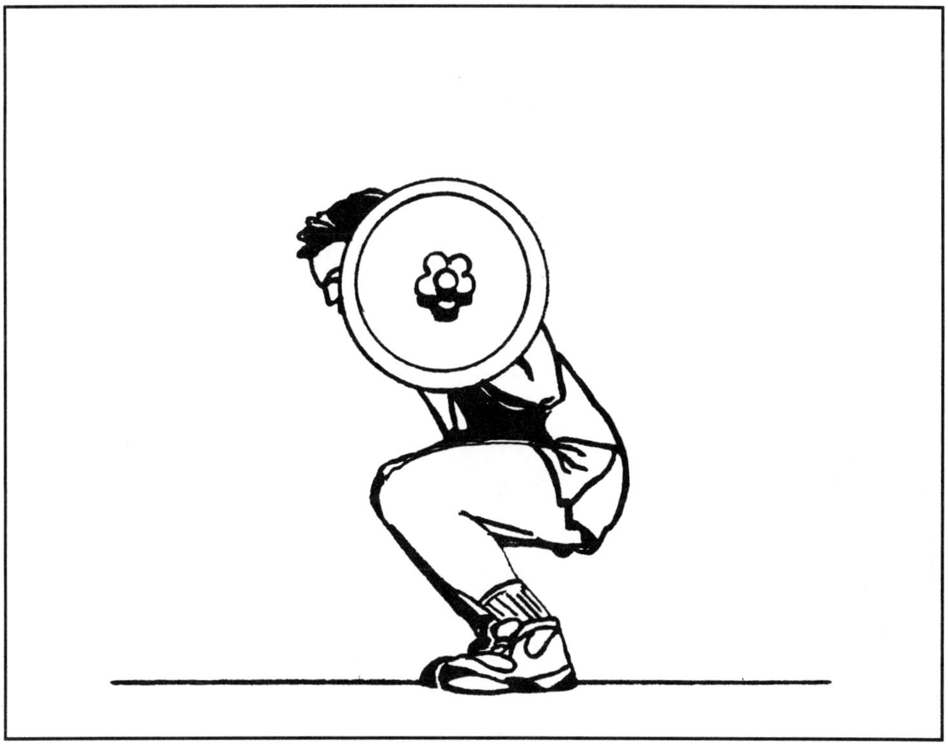

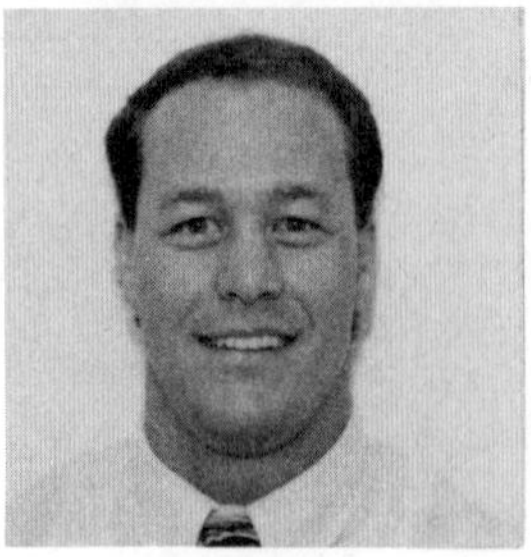

Author Jason L. Dragoo received his degree in Biological Sciences/Sports Medicine from California Polytechnic State University in San Luis Obispo, CA. This text is a result of six years of intensive research in the field of Sports Medicine with emphasis in the physiology of exercise and effects of athletic competition on young athletes. Dragoo's commitment to academic excellence is indicated by his list of academic awards, which include graduation in the top 1% of CPSU and selection as the top science student of his school. The author also competed in intercollegiate football, which gave him valuable insight in Sports Medicine from an athlete's point of view.

Dragoo also has extensive experience in amateur coaching, orthopedics, physical therapy, exercise physiology and athletic training. A summation of the knowledge acquired from his aforementioned experiences is captured in this text.

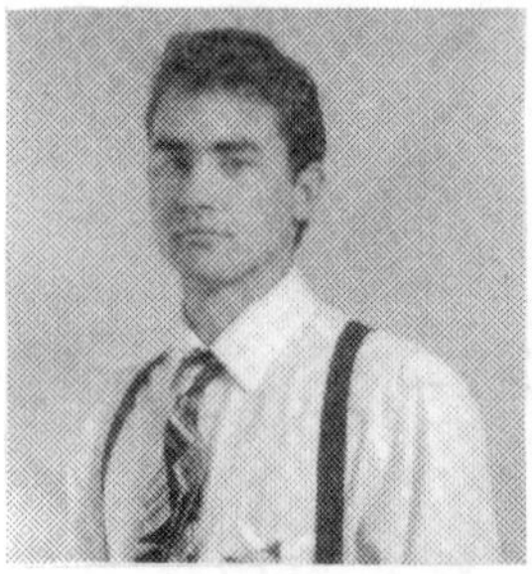

Illustrator Torey J. Arvik received his degree in Biological Sciences at California Polytechnic State University, San Luis Obispo. Besides his scientific study, Arvik has pursued an education in art. He has illustrated many other medically oriented projects, including an anatomy workbook. His dedication to both art and science has enhanced his expertise in illustration. For information on illustration services write: En Vivo Illustrations, P.O. Box 586, Applegate, CA 95703.